The Psychiatric Interview

**Dedicated to
Mary and William**

The Psychiatric Interview

Saxby Pridmore, MB, BS, BMedSc, DPhysio, MD, FAFPHM, FRANZCP

*Clinical Professor of Psychiatry, University of Tasmania and
Clinical Director of Psychological Medicine, Royal Hobart Hospital, Tasmania,
Australia*

harwood academic publishers
Australia • Canada • France • Germany • India • Japan
Luxembourg • Malaysia • The Netherlands • Russia
Singapore • Switzerland

Copyright © 2000 OPA (Overseas Publishers Association) N.V.
Published by license under the Harwood Academic Publishers imprint, part of
The Gordon and Breach Publishing Group.

Amsteldijk 166
1st Floor
1079 LH Amsterdam
The Netherlands

British Library Cataloguing in Publication Data

A catalogue record for this book is available from the British Library.

ISBN 90-5823-106-2   (soft cover)

Contents

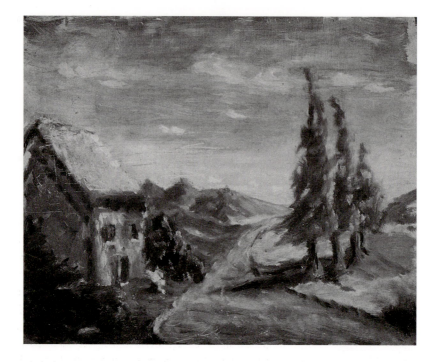

This painting was by Rosemary McGrath, daughter of Joseph and Dame Enid Lyons. Joseph was Prime Minister of Australia (1932-37) and Dame Enid was the first woman member of the Commonwealth of Australia Parliament (1943-51). Rosemary suffered schizoaffective disorder and spent many years in psychiatric hospitals. This picture, in which she used only black and shades of grey, was painted during a depressed phase.

Introduction

The aim of this book is to provide a structure and practical advice for clinicians who must conduct diagnostic interviews in psychiatry and related fields. The diagnostic interview is a single cross-sectional picture. When significant psychopathology is detected, the diagnostic interview is the beginning of management, and as with the foundations of a building, the importance of a solid job at the beginning cannot be over-emphasised. There is only one first interview between a patient and a particular clinician. That interview changes things. At future interviews the patient will not be as apprehensive, the signs and symptoms will not be as crisp and the clinician will not be as open to the range of possibilities.

Psychiatry is complex and evolving. An early task is to know what is and what is not a psychiatric problem.

Psychiatry and mental disorder

Psychiatry is a specialised field of medicine concerned with prevention, diagnosis, treatment and research of mental disorders. Mental disorders are behavioural or psychological syndromes that are associated with distress or disability (impairment in functioning).

It is important that people experiencing normal reactions are not classified as suffering from a mental disorder. Conditions that may resemble disorders appear in circumstances of loss. If a child dies (for example) the parents will suffer great sadness and may not be able to function in their usual way for some time. This is a normal reaction. It is also important to ensure that eccentricity and religious or unpopular political beliefs are not taken to be mental disorders. As recently as a decade ago, in some parts of the world people with social problems, particularly loneliness and homelessness, were offered care in psychiatric hospitals. Unless their problems have a psychiatric underpinning, such people no longer get a psychiatric bed and have correctly become the responsibility of other services.

Homosexuality and unusual sexual practices rate a special mention. If these bring no distress to the individual involved, they are not regarded as mental disorders. If they do bring distress the term mental disorder can be applied. If sexual or any other behaviour (including domestic violence) brings distress to victims, police and social workers should be involved.

The biopsychosocial model

The biopsychosocial model is useful in our understanding of the probable causes and best current management of many mental disorders. At this point, the causes of most mental disorders have not been fully determined and while some helpful treatments are available, we have few, if any, cures. Physical conditions such as bacterial pneumonia have cures, but most mental disorders, like arthritic and cardiac disorders, are chronic conditions for which we offer relief of symptoms.

The term biopsychosocial is made up of two part-words and one complete word and reminds us to consider all of these areas when dealing with patients. (This model can be usefully applied to patients with any disorder, not just those with psychiatric disorders; for example, back pain is often treated surgically without due consideration of broader and often the primary aetiological aspects of the case.)

The first syllable (bio) refers to the biological (physical) parts of the individual. This means all of the organs of the individual. In psychiatry, the brain is most commonly the organ of interest. This is demonstrated when a person suffers frontal lobe damage – after the injury there may be lack of energy and interest, neglect of personal hygiene, use of bad language and violent outbursts. When macroscopic brain changes can be detected, the term organic mental disorder is applied.

The physical structure of the brain must also be considered at the molecular, or synaptic, level. There is strong evidence that schizophrenia is associated with excessive dopamine transmission and that depressive disorders are associated with insufficient serotonin and noradrenalin transmission at certain synapses.

It is also necessary to consider the operation of other organs of the body, as pathology in some may lead to abnormality in the brain, at the synaptic level, which in turn may result in mental symptoms or disorders. The thyroid gland is an example. Both over-activity and under-activity may result in severe depression.

A genetic contribution to many mental disorders has been demonstrated and represents a major biological factor.

The role of drugs must be considered. These are physical agents that act at the synaptic level and may produce mental disorders. Examples include medical drugs such as prednisolone, which may produce mania, and propranolol, which may produce depression. Non-medical drugs such as cocaine and alcohol may also result in severe mental disorders, ranging from transient psychosis to dementia.

Physical treatments for mental disorders include psychiatric drugs and electroconvulsive therapy (ECT), both of which influence gene expression and thereby modify intracellular and synaptic structure and function.

The 'psycho' part of the term biopsychosocial refers to the psychological aspects of the individual. Two factors must be considered – the individual's personality and circumstances. Personality can be taken to mean the psychological composition (strengths, weaknesses and other psychological features) of the individual. Second, the recent events of importance to the individual. We know that loss can bring psychological distress (or psychological pain). In some individuals, but not all, severe loss (of a child, for example) may be associated with the onset of a mental disorder. It is believed that those who develop a mental disorder following loss have a constitutional (often genetic) vulnerability. Complicating the picture, psychological experiences may result in physical changes in the brain. [The brains of rats that have been exposed to learning situations have heavier and thicker cortices than those which have not had those experiences (Greenough, 1985) and hippocampal atrophy occurs in humans following traumatic events (Bremner, 1999).]

Psychological techniques may be the sole treatment of some mental disorders and are important to some degree in the treatment of all mental disorders. Psychological treatments include counselling, behavioural therapy and psychotherapy. There are many forms. They all include regular meetings between the patient and a therapist, usually over a period of months or even years. Drugs are avoided if possible and recovery results from psychological events (thoughts and other experiences) which occur during and between therapy sessions.

The 'social' part of the term biopsychosocial refers to the social aspects of the life of the individual. The social environment is important in the way we all think, feel and behave. It is well known that having a large spectator crowd cheering a team on to victory can have a profound influence on performance. In a community where children are highly valued, it can be expected that the loss of a child will be deeply distressing to the parents. However, in such a community the support and sympathy of others can help to ease the pain of bereaved parents. The lower importance placed on female children in some cultures has been reflected in differences in thinking, feeling and behaviour between the sexes.

Social factors are used in treatment, most clearly in group therapy. In this form of therapy a group of patients, often with similar problems, comes together with a therapist to talk about and explore members' disorders and themselves. Many elements are thought to be important in such therapy, including gaining confidence in dealing with groups of people, the experience of acceptance by a group and the beneficial effect of social support and encouragement.

Social factors also operate when the family is involved in the treatment and rehabilitation of a patient with a mental disorder. Because of the power of social factors, families and others (such as teachers) are involved whenever possible.

Classification and diagnosis

Large, disorganised bodies of information are difficult to understand, describe and discuss with other people. Classification, where facts are put into certain categories or boxes, makes dealing with complicated information a bit easier. The categories of disease are the diagnoses.

A diagnosis is reached after a careful history has been taken and the patient has been examined. Special investigations may prove the diagnosis, as for example in gout. But for some diagnoses, such as schizophrenia, there are no confirmatory tests.

In other branches of medicine there may be a host of physical signs – fever, swelling, tenderness, erythema, tremor, altered muscle tone – which usually assist a great deal in forming the diagnosis. In mental disorders, the physical signs – loss of affect, posturing, echopraxia – can also influence the diagnosis, but they occur less commonly, are more subtle and, in general, are less useful.

In psychiatry, the history may contain characteristic features which may be very helpful. For example, when there are delusions (false beliefs) present, the patient who believes he is guilty of a serious crime is probably suffering a depressive disorder, while the patient who believes others are guilty of serious crimes is probably suffering a paranoid disorder.

In all forms of medicine, the clinical diagnosis is based on a set of signs and symptoms, which regularly occur together. Most diagnoses carry aetiological information, as in post-traumatic stress disorder (PTSD) or prognostic information (such as in Huntington disease).

The diagnosis may sometimes carry pathophysiological information, as in phenylketonuria, but as occurs in cardiology, where a complete understanding of arrhythmias is lacking, in psychiatry, the exact pathophysiology of many disorders remains to be determined.

Around the world there are two widely used diagnostic systems – *The International Classification of Diseases*, 10th Edition (ICD 10) published by the World Health Organisation, and *The Diagnostic and Statistical Manual*, 4th Edition (DSM IV) published by the American Psychiatric Association. These are similar. In this book I use terms which are common to both systems.

The continuum of care

Making the diagnosis is an early step in care. Most psychiatric disorders are chronic in nature and with the diagnosis, a lifetime of care begins. It is necessary to bring about remission, but comprehensive and integrated follow-up must also be arranged. It is often necessary to involve social workers and psychologists, the patient's relatives, the general practitioner and the community psychiatric nurse, in addition to the psychiatrist.

An Introduction to Psychiatric Assessment

A complete assessment is the point at which good care begins. It reveals the nature and extent of the mental disorder. It may be supplemented by information from relatives, friends and others, and sometimes confirmed by special medical and psychological tests. However, even before supplementation or confirmation, a thorough initial psychiatric examination allows the crafting of an early management plan.

These pages offer some advice, but it must be understood that reading guidelines is not a substitute for experience. Clinicians can only improve their skills by examining patients, and they should take every opportunity to do so.

Comparisons can be drawn between the medical and psychiatric examinations. Both are composed of two parts – history taking, in which the clinician verbally explores the complaint and related information, and an examination in which the clinician searches for other evidence of a disorder (in medicine this is called the physical examination and in psychiatry it is called the mental state examination).

The physical examination begins with observation, and is followed by palpation, auscultation and other techniques. The mental state examination is mainly observation – there are times when it is necessary to examine the tone of a limb to determine whether side-effects of medication are present, or to place a limb in a certain position to determine whether a certain mental disorder (catatonia) is present, or to otherwise have contact with the patient, but these are relatively uncommon.

In addition to a comprehensive history and a careful mental state examination, the assessment of the psychiatric patient must also include a thorough physical examination. Some patients who present with psychiatric symptoms actually have physical disorders which mimic psychiatric disorders and which require treatment by medical or surgical rather than psychiatric methods (examples include space occupying lesions, thyroid disease, syphilis and human immunodeficiency virus (HIV), and psychiatric disorders may be compounded and sustained by medical disorders (for example, when a long-standing depressive disorder becomes unresponsive to treatment due to the recent onset of hypothyroidism – as may happen as a result of lithium therapy).

General approach

All patients have a right to be treated with respect and kindness. All psychiatric examinations and investigations must be conducted in privacy. Make sure the patient can understand what is being said – this means speaking clearly, and in the appropriate language. The clinician must introduce him/herself or be introduced to the patient, so that the patient can identify the clinician by name. Patients should be addressed by name and they should be given ample opportunity to respond to questions. During, or at the end of the interview, the patient must be given the opportunity to ask questions and the clinician must answer these as fully as possible.

In the psychiatric examination there is a place for both specific questions and open-ended questions. A specific question is one where you ask for a specific piece of information – the answer may be "yes" or "no" (such as, "Are you married?") or similarly precise information (such as, "How many children do you have?").

Open-ended questions usually do not have short, factual answers. They often require the patient to give an opinion and may thereby give the clinician access to the patient's private thoughts and feelings. Open-ended questions give few, if any, clues as to how they should be answered and are thus more likely to reveal disorder in the form and content of thought. Questions may be made more open by making them more vague. This should not be taken too far, for the more open or vague questions become, the more difficult they become, and the less likely the patient is to offer a useful answer – opting instead for an "I don't know/what do you mean?" style of response.

In taking a psychiatric history the clinician must ask both specific and open-ended questions. The relative proportions vary from one interview to another, depending on many factors, the most important being the mental state of the patient. It is not possible to give strict rules. Consider, for example, interviewing paranoid patients; some will be prepared to answer specific, factual questions, but others will find this too threatening as the style may suggest to them a police or military interrogation. On the other hand, some will be prepared to answer open questions, freely expressing delusions, while others will not, feeling they are exposing their secrets or incriminating themselves.

A thorough assessment calls for a large amount of demographic information (such as age, occupation, place of residence, marital status, number of children). This is recorded at the beginning of the written account of the assessment. It may be convenient to gather it all at the beginning of the interview – the clinician can then relax and not be concerned that these facts may be overlooked. However, because some patients find answering a lot of factual questions threatening or uncomfortable (this can be reminiscent of an interrogation), it may be better to begin by asking only a few demographic details such as the name and place of residence and then going into some general conversation, perhaps about the weather, then moving on to the presenting complaint, and picking up the rest of the demographic data as the opportunity arises. It is not uncommon for psychiatric patients to talk for a time and then become unable to continue. This may be because they have a limited amount of energy and can function in a 'normal' manner for a time, but when this energy is used, they lapse into a non-communicative state. It may be because they become fearful or focused on their private thoughts or feelings. If there is only a short time to gather diagnostically useful information, it is better spent on getting the patient's account of the presenting complaint and details of the way he/she is feeling and thinking, than on gathering factual information which will be available from the records or a family member.

It is often useful to alternate or at least intersperse specific and open-ended questions. For example, when the answer to a specific question suggests there is important information below the surface, immediately ask an open question. Such as:

Question. "Do you feel guilty, at all?"

Answer. "Well.......a little."

The examiner could then ask, "Can you please tell me about that?"

Thus, the 'closed' question yields a piece of apparently hard information and creates an opportunity for an open question, which reveals more of the patient's mental life.

Another useful technique for gaining access to the patient's mental life can be to ask for explanations. For example:

Question. "Why did you come into hospital?"

The patient has often been brought in by relatives and is not aware of his/her need for help. In such circumstances, the answer may be, "I don't know" or, "My family misunderstood what I did/said".

A follow-up question, "Well, why do you think you were brought to hospital?", or, "Well, why do you think they misunderstood?" may immediately tap into important material.

The Psychiatric History

The order in which the history is obtained and arranged in the record is, to a large degree, a matter of individual choice. For example, some choose to have a separate heading for 'Social Development' while others will place this information under the heading of 'Personal History' or 'Personality'; data relating to school life can be dealt with under a single heading, or separated out under social, educational and personality headings. Also, many psychiatrists alter the arrangement of the components of the history from one case to another – no two cases are exactly the same and a modified format may best demonstrate the significant facts of particular cases. In general, more time and space will be devoted to childhood matters in the non-psychotic than in the psychotic disorders. The following is a general outline only.

Demographic data

1. Name
2. Age
3. Religion
4. Race
5. Marital Status – single, married, divorced, widowed
6. Children – number, names, ages, live with or elsewhere
7. Education – elementary, secondary, trade, university
8. Employment Status – employed, unemployed, pensioner
9. Housing – flat, house, city, village, renting, owner

The demographic data are of great importance. They immediately give some diagnostic clues and suggest aetiological factors. These early impressions must be confirmed, but they give a starting place. For example, a 19-year-old university student who has stopped attending classes and has found no other form of employment is more likely to be suffering from schizophrenia than an anxiety disorder; a 55-year-old manufacturing company owner who has not been to work for three weeks is more likely to be suffering from depression than schizophrenia.

The demographic data also help in the understanding of the patient: the tasks he or she faces, the social supports which are likely to be available, the aspirations held, and the resources possessed. Such knowledge helps us in judging prognosis and planning treatment. For example, a 34-year-old married mother of four from a small village who attempts to hang herself, may be managed differently from a single 17-year-old girl experiencing a relationship breakdown from the same village, who also attempted to hang herself.

The presenting complaint

It can be argued that the term 'Presenting Complaint' is not always appropriate for psychiatry. The patient may not have presented themselves but may have been presented to the clinician by others, and may deny the existence of a 'complaint', vigorously asserting that he or she is 'perfectly well'. However, the term is used throughout medicine (including with unconscious patients who also neither present themselves nor offer a complaint) and is established in psychiatry. Minor terminological difficulties serve to illustrate the differences between physical medicine and psychiatry.

An account of the reasons for the presentation should be obtained from: the patient; a relative; and the referral source (which may include the police in the case of patients brought for assessment against their wishes).

It is acceptable to record the presenting complaint as a verbatim account – 'The patient said, "I heard all these murderers talking about how they are going to kill me with golden machetes"'. This form of reporting gives the flavour of the presenting complaint, but it should not be used exclusively as such accounts become very long and complicated. Technical language is a way of summarising information – thus, after exploring the above presenting complaint and clarifying the phenomena it may be possible to state: 'The patient presented complaining of auditory hallucinations. He heard three male voices plotting to kill him with golden machetes. He has the secondary delusion that his life is in danger'.

History of the presenting complaint

It may not be necessary to create a separate heading, but details of how long the complaints have been present must be included in the history.

Psychiatric disorders often develop slowly and symptoms are often not recognised in the early stages – thus, questions should be asked about

· when the patient last functioned normally
· when the patient was last well, and
· what was the first sign of change.

These are different versions of much the same question, but subtly different questions are sometimes necessary to get a clear picture of a situation.

As well as achieving longitudinal completeness, it is also necessary to get the full breadth of the history. This means asking about recent changes or symptoms which the patient may not automatically report. The presenting complaint will suggest some questions, for example, if the patient has attempted hanging and depressive disorder is suspected, in addition to mood, it is necessary to ask about changes in sleep, appetites and energy.

The following list of questions should be considered. It may not be appropriate to ask all of these of all patients.

· Changes in sleep – difficulty getting off to sleep (initial insomnia); waking in the middle of the night then getting back to sleep (middle insomnia); waking more than two hours earlier than usual and being unable to get back to sleep (early morning waking); disturbed sleep; waking unrefreshed; and excessive sleep.
· Changes in appetite (for food, sex, etc.) – any changes need to be quantified – weight loss or gain, increase or decrease in alcohol intake, alteration in the frequency of sexual relations.
· Changes in mood – depressed, sad, unhappy, fearful, worried, happy, elated, heightened sense of spirituality (closer to God).
· Changes in energy – increased or decreased.
· Changes in interest in social contact – increased or decreased.
· Changes in thought content – new or unusual thoughts, new secrets which other people might not believe, suspicious behavior or persecution by others, repetitive thoughts which cannot be ignored (particularly clever thoughts which will solve problems or make a lot of money).
· Changes in the experience of thinking – sensation of thinking being more difficult, slower or mixed-up, sensation of thinking being faster, easier or more efficient.
· New perceptions – hearing, seeing, touching, smelling.
· New physical symptoms – pains, constipation, poor vision, fits, headache, muscular weakness, loss of consciousness.

Personal history

The personal history is an account of the events in the life of the patient to the present time. As mentioned, this material can be arranged according to choice. The following is one alternative.

Birth and early development

The personal history may include information from the time before birth, where this significantly influenced the world into which the baby was born – for example, if this was an unwanted pregnancy or if the father was absent at the time of birth. Medical factors such as maternal starvation or accident during pregnancy must also be recorded.

Where the mother is available or this information is otherwise retrievable, the following are recorded: the manner of birth (vaginal or caesarean); any complications or evidence of anoxia. The early development including age at which the patient first spoke and walked, comparisons with siblings and any evidence of delays or precocity.

Family

The family history gives an account of the relationships the patient experienced. It is important to have knowledge of the following.

1. Who raised the patient.
2. Was there an adult of both sexes in the home.
3. Were either of the parents away from the home for long periods.
4. Were either, neither or both parents emotionally close to the patient.
5. How many children were there in the family and what were their names.
6. Where did the patient come in the sib-ship and what were the age differences.
7. With which of the siblings did the patient have the closest emotional relationship.
8. How would the patient describe each parent.
9. How would the patient describe the family life of his or her early years – warm, frightening, etc.

School

The school history offers valuable information. During the school years, students must function in different roles in standard settings, over an extended period of time. Thus, much objective data is available and performance patterns can be evaluated.

Patients can be asked the following questions, first in relation to primary school life and then in relation to secondary school life.

1. How did you perform scholastically with lessons and tests? (Most primary school lessons and tests are within the ability of most students. A history of having found these difficult may suggest intellectual disability. Alternatively, it may suggest the home life was very disorganised.)
2. How did you get along with the other students? (Most primary school students have at least some friends. A history of having had few friends or of being very isolated are harbingers of future difficulties. Avoidant or schizoid traits or any mental disorder manifesting at this early stage will have severe effects on development.)
3. How did you get along with the teachers? (Most primary school students have a satisfactory relationship with teachers. A history of shyness or conflict with primary school teachers suggests the early onset of difficulties with authority figures.)

Secondary school life is more complex. The lessons and tests are more difficult. Intellectual disability may become more apparent, but lack of scholastic success may occur for a variety of reasons (including difficulties at home and the emergence of personality or mental disorder).

Much may be learnt by asking about the attitudes and behaviour of friends (this allows patients to talk freely about conduct disorder in the group to which the they belonged, membership of which requires similar activities).

A history of having had friends in primary school but not in secondary school suggests a change consistent with early psychotic disorder. A history of having few friends in primary school but belonging to a group in secondary school may suggest a favourable maturation or if the group is in fact a gang, the emergence of histrionic or antisocial traits.

Difficulty with authority figures is more common in the adolescent years, but students who have sustained difficulties with secondary school teachers may have developed patterns which will apply throughout life.

Obsessional individuals may not have had a large group of friends but will usually have done well in lessons and tests throughout school.

Employment

The employment history gives a sequential account of the ability to perform a demanding adult function. It is important to obtain a complete account of:

· the type of work pursued;
· the dates of employment (starting and leaving); and
· the name of each employer.

It is also important to determine the reason for leaving each employer, and how much difficulty the patient experienced in finding the next position. The dates of employment will give the length of any periods of unemployment. If the patient claims to have had an extensive work history, it can be expected (in the absence of a paranoid state) that a list of names of employers can be given. Inability to provide such a list with a fair degree of facility suggests cognitive or factual difficulties, or fleeting contact.

Sexual, reproductive and cohabitation history

These are separate subjects, but may be grouped together to reduce the number of separate headings.

The complete sexual history includes the answers to the following questions (among others).

1. What was the attitude of the parents to sexual intimacy?
2. Did the patient ever see the parents naked?
3. How did the patient learn about sexual intimacy?
4. When was the menarche?
5. When did the patient first masturbate?
6. When and with whom was the first sexual encounter?
7. Has there been incest, rape or domestic violence?
8. Has there been homosexual contact?
9. What is the current sexual orientation?
10. How satisfactory is the patient's sex life?

Reservation – Sexual matters are among the most sensitive personal issues. While the answers to the above questions form part of a complete sexual history, the clinician may need to exercise judgement. The facts may be interwoven with fear, shame, disgust and other powerful emotions. In cases where the sexual history is probably of less relevance, such as with an acutely psychotic middle-aged patient with a long history of psychosis, it is acceptable to truncate the sexual history, at least during an acute exacerbation. In the case of individuals for whom the sexual history is of probable importance, such as a patient presenting with impotence, it may be advisable to proceed slowly and allow the patient–clinician relationship to strengthen before obtaining all necessary details.

The reproductive history includes the answers to the following questions (among others).

1. Has the patient reproduced?
2. If no to 1., have there been attempts and are there regrets?
3. If yes to 1., dates and details of births?
4. If yes to 1., what relationship does the patient now have with the off-spring?
5. In the case of women who have reproduced, was there evidence of post partum mental disorder?
6. Is the patient using contraception?
7. Does the patient wish to reproduce in the future?

Reservation – Reproductive history may be another sensitive area, especially where there has been illegitimate pregnancy of which other family members are unaware, still-birth or infertility due to earlier sexually transmitted disease. It will be necessary for clinicians to exercise judgement.

The cohabitation history is an account of the names and dates during which the patient lived in a permanent or semi-permanent sexual relationship with another (of either sex). The events of the end of relationships and the length of time between relationships are important.

Reservation – The clinician may need to exercise judgement.

Past medical and psychiatric history

Record serious medical illness/injury which may have impaired the individual's development, either by reducing opportunities, for example, as in the case of severe asthma, or by directly affecting brain function as may occur in head injury.

Record, in detail, any past psychiatric treatment.

Family medical or psychiatric history

First ask about any known family medical or psychiatric disorders, then enquire specifically about the past and present medical and psychiatric health of grandparents, parents, uncles, aunts and cousins. Ask about suicide, alcohol abuse and convictions (as these may be variants of mood disorder). Ask whether any relatives spent time in a psychiatric hospital.

Personality

An assessment of personality depends on history and observation. Thus, it sits uneasily astride the psychiatric history and the mental state examination. An assessment of personality may sometimes lead directly to a diagnosis (of personality disorder), but will always lead to predictions of behaviour.

Personality is a consistent pattern of perceiving and responding to the world and its challenges. Past predicts future behaviour.

Traits

It is important to determine the patient's:

1. predominant attitudes toward him or herself, other people, material objects and institutions;
2. ability to and attitude towards planning for the future;
3. ability/attitude to sustained effort;
4. ability to tolerate frustration;
5. ability to trust and sustain relationships;
6. coping style – forceful, seductive, methodical;
7. capacity for emotional warmth;
8. psychological mindedness (the ability to understand events from the psychological perspective);
9. superego development (internalised values or conscience);
10. alexithymia (Sifneos, 1996) is a concept not yet applied throughout psychiatry. If confirmed by further work it may have wider application. The word means 'without words to describe emotions'. It is proposed that there are people who have 'difficulty in describing or being aware of their emotions'. There are hypotheses that have alexithymia resulting from a range of causes, including neurobiological abnormality, repressive mechanisms and defective social learning.
    It is further proposed that if people are unaware or unable to describe their emotions, they may respond to stressful situations in an unexpected manner. An example may be the individual with a borderline personality who has a limited emotional repertoire and feels only the extremes of 'good' and 'bad'. It may follow that when feeling bad, such an individual may respond with anger and a physical act such as self-injury. Another example may be the individual who is unaware of, or unable to express, emotional distress who develops chronic pain.
    Thus, in the examination process it may be important to make an assessment of the individual's awareness of, and ability to express their emotions. This will be revealed by the individual's account of his or her response to previous life events and response in the interview situation. Also, alexithymic individuals may focus on facts, details and external event, act stoically and have a limited fantasy life.
    It may be important to be aware of the presence alexithymia as this may influence the amount and type of information that can be obtained from the diagnostic interview. The same may be said for all personality fea-

tures (e.g., obsessionality, shyness, irritability, etc), but alexithymia has been given special mention here because it is less well understood and less widely described.

It is necessary to distinguish between trait and state features. When certain states exist, such as episodes of mood disorder, certain features arise as a result of the state. These will disappear when the state remits. Care must be taken not to mistake these state features for personality traits (which are relatively enduring characteristics). Examples include isolative behaviour in depressed individuals which can be mistaken for an avoidant personality trait, and entitled behaviour in mood elevated individuals which can be mistaken for evidence of a narcissistic trait (Figure 1).

Sources of information

There are four main sources of information regarding personality.

1. **Personal history** – The personal history has already been described. It gives factual data regarding many aspects of the patient's behaviour.
2. **The Patient's opinion** – The patient's opinion is extremely valuable. It may reflect the opinion of others, in which case it may demonstrate a degree of self-awareness; it may conflict with the opinion of others, in

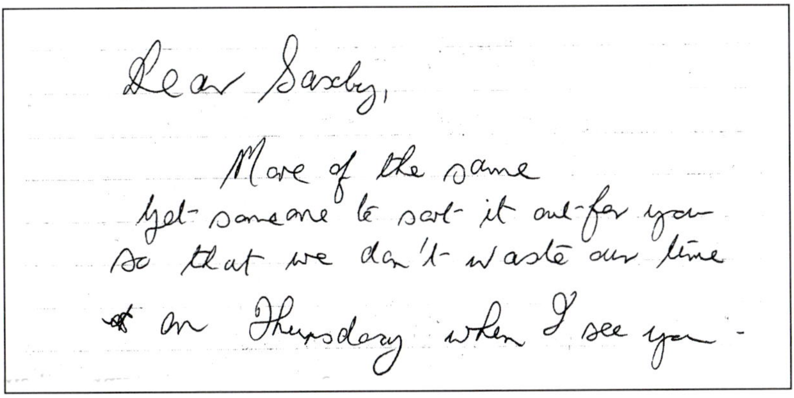
Dear Saxby,
More of the same
Get someone to sort it out for you
so that we don't waste our time
on Thursday when I see you -

Figure 1. This cover note was written by an ordinarily sedate, elderly woman who suffered mania. During acute episodes she would write prolifically and send or bring her doctor rambling letters of up to twenty pages. The above note was attached to one such letter.

Disinhibition was demonstrated in her uncharacteristic use of her doctor's christian name – a departure from their usual arrangement. There was also grandiosity in her words, 'Get someone to sort it out for you so that we don't waste our time…'. This is a state feature and not the entitlement observed in narcissistic personality disorder.

which case it may indicated inaccuracy on one side (and thereby raise further questions).

The patient should be asked to:

· give an account of his or her own personality, attitudes, strengths and weaknesses. This may or may not reveal self-awareness; and

· predict what others would say of him or her if they were asked the same questions. This may reveal paranoid, hostile/aggressive or insecure characteristics.

3. **Friends'/relatives' opinions** – A friend or relative will be able to give an account based on years of real life experience. (The clinician will need to take into account that this observation cannot be totally objective, and exercise judgement.) Relatives and friends should be asked about the patient's traits as listed above (Figure 2).

4. **The interview situation** – The above personality data is based on historical reports by the patient and others, all or whom are probably untrained. The interview situation, however, gives the opportunity for first hand observation of the patient's interpersonal behaviour. In this regard the assessment of personality is similar to the mental state examination. Does the patient respond in the interview situation with appropriate decorum, does he or she display undue informality, irritability or seductiveness. Does the patient attempt to make the clinician or others responsible for his/her situation (Figure 3). Is the patient able to use humour and healthy coping skills or is there excessive use of rationalisation and denial.

The Psychobilogical Model of Personality of Cloninger (Cloninger *et al.,* 1993) deserves mention as further work may lead to this model having a profound effect in psychiatric thinking. In this theory, personality is conceptualised as the way people learn from experience and adapt their thoughts, feelings and actions. It is divided into temperament and character. Temperament refers to the automatic responses of the individual to emotional stimuli. There are four dimensions of temperament: harm avoidance, novelty seeking, reward dependence and persistence. Character refers to voluntary goals and values, which are based on concepts of self, other people and other objects. There are three dimensions of character: self-directedness, cooperativeness and self-transcendence.

In personality disorder the individual fails to take responsibility for actions and is often in conflict with others. In the Psychobiological Model of Personality, personality disorder exists where there is a deficit in character – in particular, where there is low self-directedness and cooperativeness. Features of temperament determine the type of personality disorder rather than its presence or absence. Also, depending on character

Dear Sir,

I have addressed this letter to you – PERSONALLY – because I am sure that a lot of letters do not ever make it past the Secretary's desk. I cannot even be sure that this will - but that some 'industrious' assistant will open this and not even let you see it. Well, I shall risk that – since I really do not have any choice – do I? This may eventually end up in the garbage (where probably plenty of correspondence, which takes hours – and time and money for the person concerned). This is even more regrettable – when one cannot afford to be writing in the first place (and is a Pensioner like myself – but not an aged one, so I'm not some 'little old lady' who neither knows what she is talking about – nor can make up her own mind and in incapable of making a decision, without <u>blindly</u> being dragged into accepting things). On the contrary – God gave me a mind, and a choice – in that I have a will. I will therefore <u>exercise</u> that will – and not be 'forced' to accept your blusterings, and of other people in this Government. So be-fore, you put this in the garbage (if that is what you intend to do – and I am NOT being unkind in saying that – I actually heard a politician <u>on Television</u> – some years ago say that some (probably a lot) of the mail she got – she put straight down her toilet. PLEASE READ IT. Now I know that there may be some weird letters written in this world – but this really is a demon-strably disgusting and implicating statement – to make on national television – for all and sundry to hear. It most defi-nitely makes people wonder if their mail really is given any priority or consideration. I have had a whole lot through my life impressed upon me, to confirm me in the opinion, that is some cases – it is not ...

Figure 2. This is a facsimile of half of the first paragraph of a four-page letter sent to a federal politician. It was provided to medical staff by the relatives of a patient to assist in the diagnostic process.

In the original letter there was very little space at the top and bottom of the pages, a 5 mm margin on the left and a 1 mm margin on the right of the page, and only two paragraphs per page. It was single spaced and the pitch was small. Thus, the pages are densely covered with print. Emphasis was achieved by underlining certain words and placing others in capitals.

The correspondent opens with concern that the letter may not receive due consideration from the recipient. Only one other matter is raised and this is what the correspondent describes as misplaced encouragement afforded to two minority groups.

There is no disorder in the form or content of thought as described elsewhere in this book. There is a repetitious, ponderous style with no warmth. While no paranoid delusions are present, there is intolerance and anger. The question of morality is raised and a dictionary definition given. This letter is of the type written by individuals with obsessive–compulsive personality disorder.

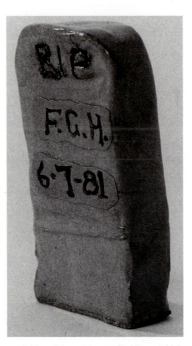

Figure 3. This ceramic model headstone was crafted by a middle-aged man with a histrionic personality disorder.

He was admitted to a psychiatric hospital with what would now be diagnosed as an adjustment disorder with depressed mood, following a failed relationship. This was at a time when such places had occupational therapy departments and the pressure to discharge patients was not as it became in later years.

Ten days after admission this patient went to the occupational therapy department and completed the first step of construction – a wet clay model of a headstone bearing the letters RIP, his own initials and a date some two weeks hence. There was concern among staff that this man planned to kill himself, but because this appeared to display attention-seeking behaviour, the model was not discussed with him. He was unobtrusively watched more closely. Subsequently, the patient dried the model in the kiln and finally, glazed and fired it again. He did not offer comment about his model but displayed it prominently at every step of construction. His condition improved, the headstone date passed and he was discharged. He left the model unclaimed in the occupational therapy department and it was thrown out a year later. The patient was alive nearly two decades later.

The important features were the dramatic and attention-seeking behaviour involved in the making of this model, and the superficiality suggested by it being forgotten.

configuration, the same temperamental configuration will lead to different outcomes. For example, where there is healthy character development, high novelty seeking may lead to a quiet life in research, while where there is low self-directedness and cooperativeness, high novelty seeking may lead to irresponsible, even criminal, behaviour.

Motivation, apathy and will

Inclusion of this section in the assessment of the psychiatric patient is controversial, but I consider it useful. It is a complicated area, incorporating philosophy and the history of ideas, which is beyond the scope of this book – but a skeleton gives some context. In ancient Greece the psyche was regarded as being composed of three parts: affect (feeling), cognition (knowing) and conation (that aspect of the mental processes having to do with volition, striving and willing). The close integration of the components of the psyche makes their separation difficult and Kaplan and Saddock (1998) places conation under the heading of motor behaviour.

Berrios (1996) sees great value in the concept of the will. He notes that toward the end of the nineteenth century it became 'a casualty of fashion' and fell from use, a fall hastened by the rise of psychoanalysis and behaviourism. Berrios and Gili (1995) state that the will was an important descriptive and explanatory concept and that removal led to a conceptual vacuum in the domain of volition which has been unsatisfactorily filled by notions of instinct, drive, motivation, etc. They contend that will remains 'central to psychiatry' and that it is relevant to personality disorder, chronic fatigue syndrome and forensic psychiatry.

Silva and Martin (1999) have made a useful contribution. They describe apathy as the diminution in motivation (observable goal-directed behaviour) relative to a person's age and culture, claiming it becomes clinically significant when severe enough to interfere with psychosocial functioning. They report that apathy occurs in a range of neuropsychiatric and medical conditions including dementia, frontal lobe syndrome, basal ganglia disease, stroke, depression and psychotic disorders. To this list it would be reasonable to add personality disorder.

Observers can agree that individuals may differ in their motivation (goal-directed behaviour) and that one individual may be highly motivated in a broad range of aspects of life, while another may be highly motivated in only one aspect (a hobby, perhaps, collecting stamps). But if the topic is approached from another direction, questions may be raised about what is energising or directing the motivation and perhaps that is the Holy Grail we should be pursuing. The question of 'will' can be similarly viewed as multilayered. First, there is the aspect of energy (Plato used the term 'bouelsis' in the discussion of will, a word which is related to boiling and exuberant) and secondly, the choice regarding how to direct that energy. Kant (1909) stated that the will 'is conceived as a faculty of determining oneself to action...' – the word 'determining' conveying a measure of choice or deciding on direction. For present purposes, consid-

eration is given only of the evidence of motivation and not to the associated issues of choice.

It is believed possible to make a statement about the amount of motivation demonstrated by a patient. There is need for caution as there is a
danger that the clinician may appear to be making a moral judgement.
Using the term 'will', for example, leads to classifications of 'strong willed'
and 'weak willed' – while technically defensible, such classifications could
expose the clinician to criticism. The term 'motivation' is a possible substitute – the patient can be placed on a continuum form 'highly motivated'
to 'lacking motivation', the latter term being more socially acceptable
than 'weak willed'. As an Apathy Evaluation Scale (Martin *et al.,* 1991) has
been created and validated, 'apathy' is also a suitable choice. Patients can
be rated from 'severely apathetic' through to 'no evidence of apathy' – it is
then possible to extend beyond that point to 'highly motivated'.

Where comment on motivation, apathy and will should appear in the
written assessment is flexible. These elements are closely related to motor
behaviour, however, they are also touched on in personal history, and
parts are included under personality. Like personality, they sits astride the
history–examination border. Therefore, it is recommended that motivation, apathy and will follow the entry on personality.

Diagnostic considerations

Many mental disorders manifest symptoms which could be included under
this heading.

Depression

Particularly in major depressive epsodes, the depressed patient may complain of loss of motivation and disabling fatiguability. This may be associated
with slowed movement and thinking (psychomotor retardation). These are
biological or vegetative features of this medical/psychiatric disorder, but
the patient may interpret them as moral or character flaws. Such a view
may accentuate self-loathing and delusions of guild. All of these symptoms, including the loss of motivation and disabling fatiguability, are
reduced by effective treatment..

Schizophrenia

Particularly in chronic schizophrenia, patients may complain of a loss of
motivation. Frequently, it is family, friends or health professionals who
make this observation. It is one of the "negative symptoms" of schizophre-

nia, others being loss of affect and poverty of thought. Such synmptoms may result in self-neglect. The "negative symptoms" result from the loss of normal functions, whereas the "positive symptoms" such as hallucinations and delusions are additions to normal experience. In schizophrenia the negative symptoms are notoriously unresponsive to treatment.

Neurasthenia and fatigue syndromes

Neurasthenia appears in the ICD-10. It is a diagnostic category which has been rejected and reinstated by different authorities at different times. The ICD-10 states that there are two main types. In one, after mental effort there is mental fatigue which "is typically described as an unpleasant intrusion of distracting associations or recollections, difficulty in concentrating, and generally inefficient thinking". In the other, after minimal physical effort there are feelings of physical weakness, muscular aches and an inability to relax. There are other symptoms, but the hallmark is the fatiguability and weakness. To make this diagnosis, one must first exclude physical or other psychiatric causes. While there is some resistance to linking fatigure syndromes with neurasthenia, no distinction is made in ICD-10.

Personality disorder

In early diagnostic classifications there was an "inadequate" personality category. Such individuals were believed to lack motivation. No such category is now recognised.

Mental State Examination

1. Appearance and Behaviour

These are difficult areas. The appearance, manners and behaviour of the patient may be of importance when there is significant deviation from that of his or her socioeconomic group. Remember that style of dress and behaviour vary with the geographic origin and socioeconomic status of the individual, and the fashion of the day. While appearance and behaviour demonstrate membership of a certain group in time and place, they may also be a means of expression of individuality, identity or independence from the group. Just as there are some people for whom fashion is a revered and practised art form (akin to sculpture) there are others who have no interest or skill in the matter. Thus, one must be alert to the many normal differences in appearance and behaviour, and be cautious in attributing differences in appearance and behaviour to mental disorder.

Appearance

Personality traits

Appearance may suggest personality traits. Collaborative data must always be obtained.

· A high degree of attention to correctness, cleanliness, tidiness and detail suggests obsessional traits. In many instances, but not always, conservatism in appearance is a feature of obsessional traits.
· A high degree of attention to fashion may suggest narcissistic traits. The above points regarding fashion and the desire to belong to a group must be considered.
· A high degree of attention to flamboyant or seductive appearance may suggest histrionic traits. Flamboyant appearance may also be a feature of the isolated eccentric or the charismatic leader.

Mental disorder

Appearance may suggest mental disorder. Collaborative data must always be obtained.

The 'omega sign' has been described on the forehead of many people suffering depression (Grenden *et al.*, 1985). The eyebrows form the bottom of the omega figure and folds pass up and laterally from the glabella (Verraguth's folds) to be joined superiorly by horizontal wrinkles. This is consistent with increased activity in the Corrugator supercilii, which draws the eyebrows down and medially and was described in Gray's Anatomy (Davies and Davies, 1962) as 'the principal muscle in the expression of suffering'.

The 'long face' has also been described in depression. The distance from the outer canthus of the eyes to the corners of the mouth has been shown to be significantly greater in those with depression than in non-depressed people, using a method of quantification of facial expression (Katsikitis and Pilowsky, 1991). This is consistent with decreased activity of the Zygomaticus major and Zygomaticus minor. Electromyographic studies have given support to the theory of increased activity in Corrugator supercilii and decreased activity in Zygomaticus minor and Zygomaticus major in depression (Carney *et al.*, 1981) (Figure 4).

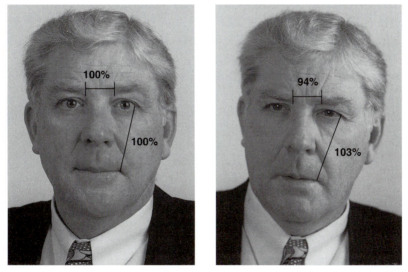

Figure 4. This is the face of an actor. On the right is a portrayal of the facies in depression. The eyebrows are drawn down and together and the omega sign and Verraguth's folds appear on the forehead. The face is 'long' in that the mouth is lower – that is, the corners of the mouth are lower, relative to the outer canthi of the eyes. The mouth is also less wide. The portrayal on the left is of a neutral, not smiling expression, for comparison.

Bizarre appearance, such as the wearing of special headgear designed to protect against radiation, is quite rare. It suggests psychosis. Less dramatic signs such as the uncharacteristic shaving of the head or wearing of religious insignia where none were worn before, may also represent acute psychosis, whether arising from a delusional system, disorganised thinking or uncomfortable feelings. Mood elevation may rarely result in bizarre appearance and behaviour (Figure 5).

Self-neglect of recent onset as when a patient presents in relatively new, expensive clothes but with food stains on the front or smelling of urine and body odour may suggest an organic disorder such as dementia, or a severe functional disorder such as retarded depression.

Self-neglect of long standing such as when a person who has had extensive dental attention evidenced by gold fillings presents with many cavities and poor oral hygiene, suggests a chronic disorder such as frontal lobe syndrome or chronic schizophrenia.

Colourful dressing as when a patient presents wearing bright prime colours may suggests mania. In such cases there may also be excessive use of jewellery, and necklaces and earrings may be wrapped around wrists or pinned to the front of the clothes.

Sombre dressing, such as the wearing of dark colours, may be a feature of depression. This is not particularly striking. It may become so in retrospect when the recovering patient begins to wear colours.

Behaviour

Marked agitation may be a feature of a young, insecure or frightened individual, an anxiety disorder, an agitated depression or a psychotic individual with persecutory delusions. When dealing with a highly agitated individual it is best to have assistance close at hand and for both the interviewer and the patient to be able to rapidly vacate the office.

Threatening or intimidating behaviour may take the form of raised voice or shouting, standing very close to or over the interviewer, as well as raising fists or hands. Such behaviour is rare. It may be demonstrated by intoxicated individuals, aggressive individuals without a psychiatric disorder, aggressive antisocial individuals and psychotic individuals with persecutory delusions. Staff must not tolerate such behaviour and must immediately leave the person or call for assistance.

Increased activity may take the form of frequent, quick, large-amplitude movements of the hands and standing to walk around, the demonstration of points with actions and unexpected leaving of the room. Where there is increased activity, the voice is often loud and the speech

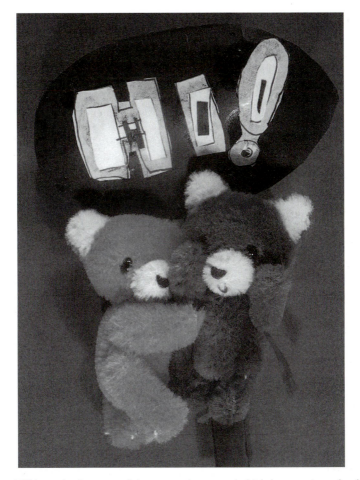

Figure 5. This construction was made by a reserved young geologist during an acute manic episode. She had been admitted to hospital but slipped away and went into a bank – where she was not a customer and was not known.

The source of the toy bears remains a mystery to all, including the patient.

At a customer desk in the bank, she made the construction. She asked the tellers for things as she required them. She first asked for scissors and cut cardboard promotional material to form the components of the sign post. She asked for colored paper from which she cut the letters. She then asked for the use of a stapler and glue to complete the work. The 'HI!' is composed of three layers of ever smaller letters, first pink, then white and finally very small black letters. In other circumstances the construction may have been more colorful, but banks stock limited creational materials.

It was surprising that this patient, who was so disorganised as to have no memory of the acquisition of the toy bears, had organisational and concentrational abilities sufficient to perform this reasonably delicate work. But in mania (and many other mental disorders), psychopathology is notoriously variable and patchy.

Once completed, this construction was carried by the patient as a greeting placard along the streets back to the hospital (where she made a gift of it to her treating doctor). For this normally demure young person, carrying this construction in public constituted bizarre appearance and behaviour.

rapid. This picture suggests mania, in which case the face is often smiling. In mania, the jovial appearance may change to anger and irritability if the patient is obstructed, as when the patient is prevented from leaving. Irrespective of obstruction, joviality is a common feature of early mania, but irritability frequently supersedes as the episode progresses. Attention deficit disorder, delirium, thyrotoxicosis, stimulant abuse and akathisia deserve consideration.

Decreased activity may take the form of sitting still with reduced hand gestures and facial movement. Decreased activity may be associated with slow movement and slow, monotonous talk (see later). When the movements are slow and the patient complains of (or admits to) the experience of slower than usual thinking the term 'psychomotor retardation' may be applied. Acute depression, chronic schizophrenia, mental retardation, hypothyroidism and Parkinsonism (idiopathic and drug induced) must be considered.

Repetitive movements include 'tics' and 'stereotypy'. Tics are sudden non-rhythmic movements (such as shoulder shrugging) or vocal productions (such as sniffing). They are involuntary but can be voluntarily suppressed. Transient tics may appear in healthy individuals at times of stress. Tics which may fluctuate in severity occur in Tourette's syndrome, obsessive compulsive disorder and attention deficit disorder. Huntington's disease and Wilson's disease must be excluded. Stereotypy is intentional, repetitive, non-functional behaviour such as body-rocking or head-banging – styreotypic movement disorder is a DSM-IV diagnosis and occurs with intellectual disability. Stereotypy is now uncommon in schizophrenia (it was once more common in this disorder).

'Echopraxia' is the term applied when the patient unconsciously copies the interviewer's movements. This is not an act of ridicule. In severe cases it is clearly present, but in less severe cases (which are much more common) it is subtle and easily missed. For example, only some movements may be replicated, the patient crossing the legs or touching the face shortly after the interviewer has done so. Echopraxia may be associated with drug intoxication, drug-induced psychosis and schizophrenia.

'Catatonic symptoms' occur when the pathological mental state is expressed in motor anomalies. They may be categorised as the following.

· 'Catatonic Stupor' in which movement ceases and the patient is unresponsive to the spoken word or even to painful stimuli. There is usually also the failure to take food or fluid. Accordingly, the life of the patient may be in danger.

· 'Catatonic Posturing' in which the patient assumes a posture which is then maintained. This might be a strange posture such as standing on one leg with the arms out sideways in the middle of the front path, but it is usually more subtle and may simply impress as an awkward or uncomfortable way to sit or stand.

· 'Catatonic Rigidity' in which a posture is maintained against the interviewer's attempts to move the limbs or the whole patient.

· 'Waxy Flexibility' in which the interviewer can change the position of the patient's limbs, and in the process the limbs feel to the interviewer as if they are made of wax. (The new posture is usually then maintained for at least a few seconds and sometimes minutes.)

Catatonic symptoms are infrequently encountered. They are most commonly associated with psychotic depression and schizophrenia (Figure 6), but are also seen in conversion and organic disorders.

Someone knocked loudly on their window, signalling me to go in their place. They seemed very angry so I didn't go in. I stopped still at the corner of Brittania St. and Melbourne Road. This was because I felt Satan was leading me into a trap if I kept on walking. I was as still as a statue. God's peace kept my mind. It started to drizzle lightly, so light that I couldn't feel the rain on my head. After a while a lady came out with her family. They were staring at me strangely. She said "What are you doing here?" I said, "God sent me."

After they went inside, I began to walk down Brittania St. Because I had been standing for about half an hour I found it extremely hard and painful to lift my feet off the ground. Finally, I got into the next street where two policemen met me. They said that six different people phoned up complaining about me. We were talking a while not getting anywhere when I heard a voice say "Go".

I later realised that the voice was trying and successful in getting me into trouble. I ran, faster than I had ever ran. After running 100 yards, I stopped. The policemen running after me was 50 yards behind and the police car was just pulling up beside me. They put me in the van. I was cold. Just then Mr. Brown my church Minister came along. He assured the policemen that I was due for a breakdown and that I was a fast runner. Even though I hadn't run fast in years.

Figure 6. This was written by a young man who suffered schizophrenia and eventually died by suicide.

When he wrote that he was as 'still as a statue' for half an hour, the patient was probably describing a period of catatonia. There is some delusional material in the first paragraph. In the second paragraph the patient describes a command hallucination to which he responded. The third paragraph has a light-hearted flavor – this may have been intentional; more probably, it is the result of disorganised thinking and affect of the type which may occur in disorganised (hebephrenic) schizophrenia.

'Self-cutting or slashing' on the arms is usually taken as an expression of suicidal intention or desire. It is mistake to attempt conclusions about the degree of psychopathology and intentions from the site and depth of the cutting. Cuts on the volar or inside of the wrist have greater potential to cause death, but the lay person may not be aware of this and thus cuts on the dorsum or outside of the forearm may represent a strong intention to die. Cuts on the volar aspect of the wrist, which sever arfteries, nerves or tendons, call for surgical intervention and suggest a major depressive or a psychotic disorder.

Self-cutting on the dorsum of the forearm, amid old scars from previous episodes may represent a maladaptive tension releasing or communication technique, and possibly a feature of personality disorder.

'Self-mutilation' is usually also achieved by cutting. It does not carry immediate risk to life and is believed to be a different phenomenon. It involves the removal of body parts such as eye, finger, penis or external ear, and cuts to the face, body or limbs. Cuts to the body may be to the breasts or genitalia. To be classed as self-mutilation, cuts to the arms and legs must be disfiguring.

Generally, self-mutilation suggests psychotic disorder. In such circumstances the act my be conducted in response to command hallucinations (Figure 7), delusion or as sudden, inexplicable, bizarre behaviour, perhaps underpinned by labile affect. Dr William Minor amputated his penis, apparently as a consequence of delusional thinking (Winchester, 1998).

Self-mutilation is not exclusive to psychosis. In recent times, self-mutilation has been fashionable in Australian prisons among non-psychotic individuals. One notorious Australian prisoner earned the nickname 'Chopper' by cutting off his external ears. Such mutilation gives a frightening appearance, but the motivation has not been researched. I have known a patient who removed fingers at different times and no diagnosis other than personality disorder could be discovered.

'Suicidal behaviour' other than cutting is not uncommon. This has usually preceded presentation, but on occasions, will occur while the patient is waiting or after assessment. It may take the form of self-hanging. In such instances, as there is rarely a strong rope to hand, the attempt may be made with a flimsy article such as a tape measure, with little prospect of causing death. Such behaviour may suggest factitious disorder or malingering. On the other hand, it may symbolise a strong desire for death, and must be evaluated.

'Bizarre or inexplicable behaviour' is uncommon. Examples from my experience include the directing of street traffic without authority, walking naked in the street with clear consciousness, and the unpremedi-

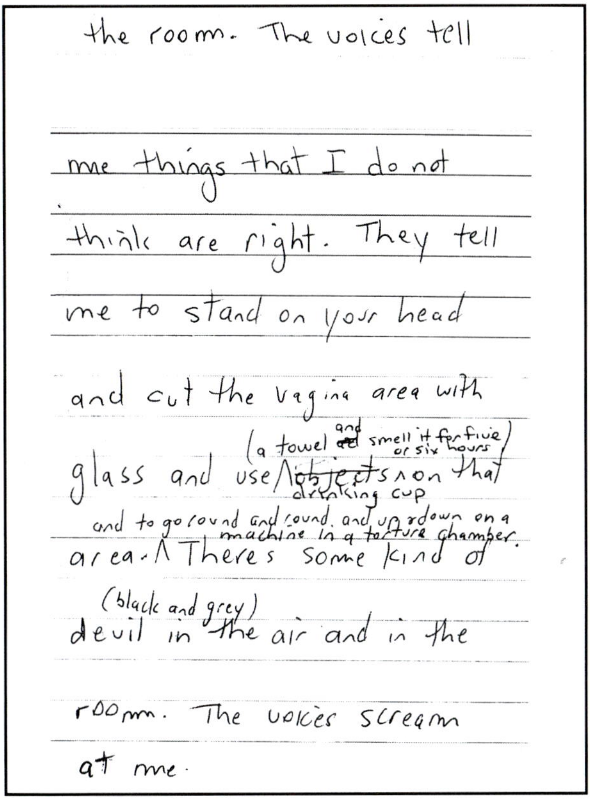

> the room. The voices tell
>
> me things that I do not
>
> think are right. They tell
>
> me to stand on your head
>
> and cut the vagina area with
>
> glass and use /objects\ on that (a towel and smell it for five or six hours) drinking cup
>
> area. /\ There s some kind of and to go round and round and up rdown on a machine in a torture chamber.
>
> devil in the air and in the (black and grey)
>
> room. The voices scream
>
> at me.

Figure 7. This is from the note-pad writings of a middle-aged woman who was suffering acute schizophrenia. Her first lines subsequently had additional smaller entries squeezed in between them.

In this example she writes that hallucinations told her to self-mutilate: "...cut the vagina area with glass..." In the next line she states "The voices scream at me". It is probable that when she failed to comply with command hallucinations (she did not think they were 'right'), they became louder and more insistent.

The subsequently added lines indicate that her vaginal area should "go round and round and up and down on a machine in a torture chamber". The thread is broken, it is not clear whether these added lines were of hallucinatory or delusional origin.

Some entries indicate formal thought disorder. For example, the addition "drinking cup" is placed after glass. It is unlikely, although possible, that "the voices" told this patient to cut her vaginal area with a drinking cup. It is likely that when she was rereading her first entry, she derailed from glass to drinking cup, and then added this detail.

"Black and grey" devils are described "in the air". This probably indicates visual hallucinations; the visual hallucinations of schizophrenia are often shadow-like and lack clear details.

Where patients are experiencing command hallucinations or delusions indicating self-mutilations, there is need for caution and active treatment.

tated fatal stabbing of a child. In each of these cases the patient was psychotic, but factitious disorder and malingering must be excluded.

2. Talk

The decision on which aspects of the mental state examination are presented under separate headings is arbitrary. Talk justifies separate consideration as it occurs in all interviews and some straightforward observations can be made. The word talk is chosen rather than 'speech', as this word is often used synonomously with thought. Talk is restricted to some of the mechanical aspects of verbal communication, articulation, volume, speed and pitch.

Articulation

The clarity with which words are spoken is the focus of attention. Dysarthria or mumbling suggests mechanical problems. Pathology may exist as upper-motor (cortical) or lower-motor (cranial nerve) lesions. Slowly progressing neurological disorders such as Huntington's disease and multiple sclerosis need to be excluded. Slurred words may also result from acute neurological damage, fatigue, sedation, acute extrapyramidal side effects of medication, dry mouth and intoxication. It has been noted that many people with chronic schizophrenia do not speak clearly; important factors may include, tardive dyskinesia, thought disorder resulting in new words, lack of practice and volition, and loss of the coodination frunction of the frontal lobes and cerebellum.

Volume

Loud talk may be a feature of mania, in which case it is a manifestation of increased energy. It may be a characteristic of an individual who wishes to make a strong impression, such as in the case of an individual with histrionic traits.

Quiet talk may be a feature of depression or the characteristic of an unassertive individual.

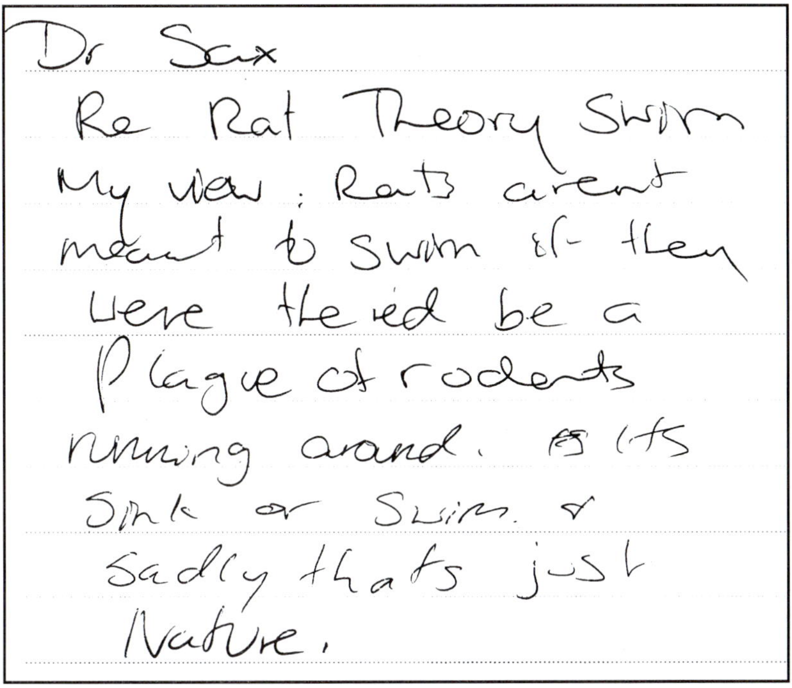

Dr Sax

Re Rat Theory Swim
My view : Rats aren't
meant to swim & if they
were there'd be a
Plague of rodents
running around. & its
Sink or Swim. &
Sadly thats just
Nature.

Figure 8. This letter was written by a middle-aged man who was suffering from mania. He was in the audience at a lecture I gave. The Porsolot Swim Test was mentioned, a laboratory test in which the time is recorded for which a rat swims in water before giving up and having to be plucked out by the scientists. It is used in the testing of antidepressant medication.

This letter was written in haste, which increased toward the end.

Speed

Rapid talk may be a feature of mania, anxiety and stimulant use (Figure 8). Slow talk may be a feature of depression, sedation or intoxication.

Pressure of speech/thought/talk

This phenomenon can be placed under different headings, and will be mentioned again in the section on Thought under the heading of flight of ideas.

With pressure of speech there is an increase in speed of talk, the voice is usually loud and the patient cannot be interrupted. Sometimes the patient will simply 'talk over' (speak louder) when the interviewer asks a question. Where there is much pressure of speech, the patient will talk when there is no one else present. Sentences may be left uncompleted, the patient passing on to different topics, there may be flight of ideas (see later) which is difficult to follow or rhyming or punning speech.

Pressure of speech is characteristic of mania, but stimulant intoxication must be excluded.

Pitch

High-pitched talk may be the result of fear, anxiety or arousal.

Constant low-pitched talk may be the result of depression or hypothyroidism.

Dysprosody is the loss of the normal melody of talk. This occurs by definition with the constant low-pitched talk of depression. However, the term is usually applied where the lack of fluctuation in pitch is a feature of chronic schizophrenia and prefrontal–mesocortical damage. In schizophrenia, dysprosody is often associated with disorder of affect. Where dysprosody is a feature of depression, it is expected to resolve with the resolution of the episode. Where it is a feature of chronic schizophrenia, dysprosody is less likely to resolve (as current treatments have minimal effect).

3. Mood

There are some features of mental state assessment on which there are divergent definitions and views. Mood is one of these.

Mood has been defined (Kaplan and Saddock, 1991) as a pervasive and sustained emotion, subjectively experienced and reported by the patient, as well as observed by others. There are four important elements in this definition. First, that mood is sustained, in the normal individual mood is usually measured in the order of hours (although environmental stimulus such as good or bad news may result in a sudden change). In mood disorder the mood is frequently sustained for months. Second, the pervasive characteristic, meaning that the influence of mood extends throughout the mental life, modifying thinking and behaviour. For example, when there is severely depressed mood, thoughts may turn to sad events and delusions of guilt, and behaviour may include suicide. Third, that mood is subjectively experienced by the patient. To be certain on this point the interviewer must ask about the patient's mood. (This part of the mental state examination, in which the patient gives information, bears a similarity to psychiatric history taking). Fourth, evidence of mood should be observable by the interviewer.

While many moods are described in literature, psychology and daily life, those of chief interest in psychiatry are sustained depression, elation, irritability and anxiety.

As mood has a subjective component, it is necessary to enquire. Questions like 'How have you been feeling in yourself/your spirits?' begin to tap into mood. The response, once clarified, must be recorded. It should be followed by a comment as to whether this is consistent with the interviewer's finding. The observations contributing to the interviewer's finding may be briefly listed.

Poems by Davina Sutton-Driscoll

The Spiral Down

I'm alive in Hell
burning inside out.
I scream without sound and
cry without the gift of tears.
Looking back I see...
a life
a smile
a dream or two.
I watch from a window
without faith or hope.
This is my final full stop.

I can barely breathe
I can't even shit without
        medication.

Lust

I want to get in a car and
drive until the world caves in.
I want to be arrested for being alive.
I want to drink tequila for morning tea and
wear nothing but purple.
I want a fabulous love affair
with no restrictions and
ice cream that isn't fattening.
I want a best friend for every day of the year
and a house with windows in every wall.
I want a world without cigarette butts and
                garlic breath
and a street where people dance on a whim.

I want to understand one thing
why socks go missing and knickers never do.

Labour For Life

I'm having contractions.
My moods are five minutes apart.
I'm calm and then contorted
I ride an escalator up and down

I need to stop the ride
get off and have a coffee.
The problem is
I'm out of money and things just
        won't slow down.

Polluted

My mind needs an enema.
Something clean to soothe the area
a bath or a shower at least
I'm dirty mentally and
I go rotten daily.

My emotions need airing.

I belong in the dirty linen trolley.

Figure 9. Ms Sutton-Driscoll is a young poet who suffers bipolar disorder. In 'The Spiral Down' and 'Polluted', she mentions the depressed mood, self-loathing, hopelessness, inability to cry and constipation of the depressed phase of bipolar disorder. In 'Labour of Life', she describes the discomfort of rapidly fluctuating feelings of sadness and happiness which may occur when a patient is recovering from an abnormal mood state (depression or mania) or passing from one abnormal mood state to another. In 'Lust', Ms Sutton-Driscoll describes subsequent feelings, energy, elation and humor, when she has passed into a hypomanic phase.

Depression

Subjective experience

A variety of words, many colloquial, may be used to describe depressed mood. These include, 'sad', 'low', 'down', 'blue', 'no good', 'not much good' and 'like shit'. The characteristic Australian response, 'not bad', can be used in a non-committal manner and can camouflage the expression of depression (Figure 9).

Some patients deny the presence of depressed mood. This may arise because of a conscious decision to hide the emotion, or in some instances the patient may not be aware of depressed mood. In such cases the prominent feature may be the inability to experience pleasure or unexplained physical pain (and terms such as smiling depression or masked depression have been applied).

Objective findings

The behaviour and talk of seriously depressed patients has already been mentioned. The clinician should record evidence of slow movements, monotonous talk, sad face, immobile face, downcast eyes and crying.

In addition to the various depressive disorders (major depressive disorder, cyclothymia, dysthymia and adjustment with depressed mood), consider common disappointment. (People with personality disorder experience frequent conflicts and disappointments.) People suffering the negative symptoms of schizophrenia may appear depressed. Physical conditions worthy of consideration include hypothyroidism and Parkinsonism (idiopathic and drug included).

Elation

Subjective experience

The patient may deny any mood symptoms either because they are not aware that the elation is pathological (in which case they may say everybody should feel the way they do) or because they enjoy the feeling and wish to avoid treatment. Others will admit to feeling 'high', 'racing/racy' and 'wonderful'. (Figure 10).

Objective findings

The behaviour and talk of elated patients has already been mentioned. The clinician should record evidence of loud, rapid talk, continuous smiling, informality, colourful dress, uninhibited talk of sex and pressure of speech.

The presence of elation suggest mania or schizoaffective disorder (mood elevated episode). Exclude stimulant use and organic mood disorder (in particular, supraspinal multiple sclerosis, pseudobulbar palsy and frontal lobe syndrome).

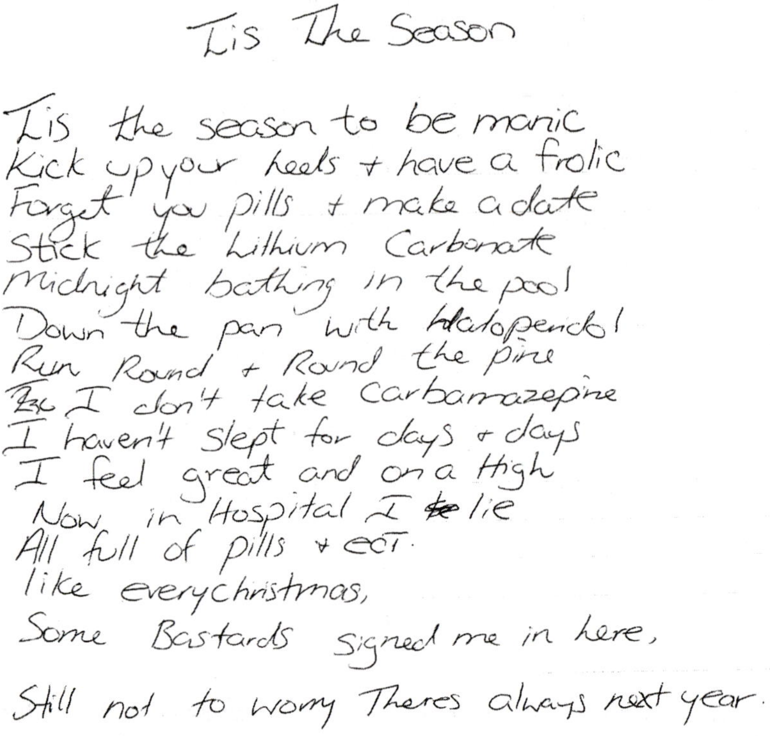

Tis The Season

Tis the season to be manic
Kick up your heels + have a frolic
Forget you pills + make a date
Stick the Lithium Carbonate
Midnight bathing in the pool
Down the pan with Haloperidol
Run Round + Round the pine
Bc I don't take Carbamazepine
I haven't slept for days + days
I feel great and on a High
Now in Hospital I lie
All full of pills + ECT.
like everychristmas,
Some Bastards signed me in here,

Still not to worry Theres always next year.

Figure 10. This was written by a young person suffering an acute manic episode. Mood elevation led to light hearted poetry. This is rhyming verse, rather than clang associations as there is an effort to get a rhythm into the lines and the rhymes have been worked out rather than have occurred automatically (pool and haloperidol). The content includes the rejection of many of the known treatments (lithium, carbamazepine, haloperidol and ECT), over-activity and sleeplessness. The patient describes mood elation – "I feel great and on a high". There is only one possible suggestion of irritability, when those who initiated compulsory detention are referred to as "Bastards", followed immediately by the euphoric "Still not to worry Theres always next year".

Irritability

Subjective experience

It is common to deny irritability and to justify the evidence of irritability on the grounds that any normal person would be annoyed by the interviewer's persistent and stupid questions. Others will admit to feeling 'crabby', 'snappy', 'angry', 'out of sorts' and 'hard to get along with'. Many will remark that irritability is an unpleasant experience.

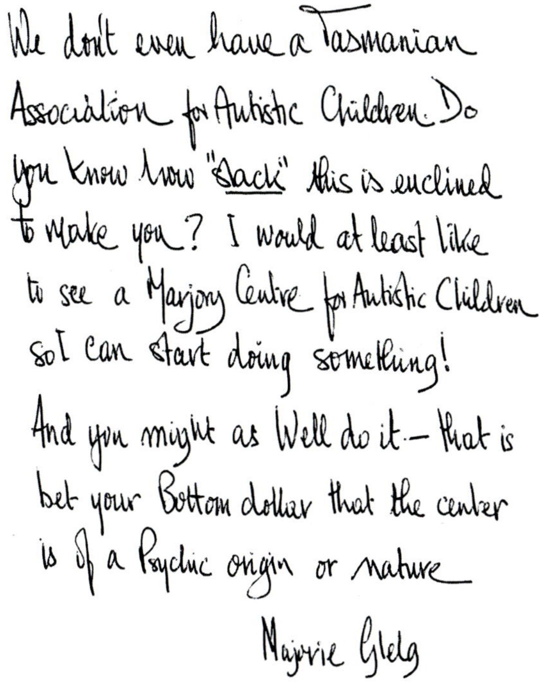

We don't even have a Tasmanian
Association for Autistic Children. Do
you know how "<u>Sick</u>" this is enclined
to make you? I would at least like
to see a Marjory Centre for Autistic Children
so I can start doing something!

And you might as Well do it — that is
bet your Bottom dollar that the center
is of a Psychic origin or nature

Marjorie Gielg

Figure 11. This letter was written to me when I was in a senior administrative position by a female patient of another psychiatrist. It was known that this person was the patient of another psychiatrist because she mentioned the fact in another letter. No other information is known about this person.

There are many grammatical errors and the word 'psychic' is used where the word 'psychiatric' would have been more appropriate. The language and educational background of the correspondent is unknown, so it is impossible to judge whether there is any superimposed thought disorder. (The hand writing, however, suggests experience in this form of communication.)

It is assumed that the correspondent is suffering a manic episode. First, there is an abrupt opening and ending, with neither the usual introductory remarks nor wishes for further discussion. Second, there is grandiosity, the facility to be named after the correspondent. Finally, there is irritability, the correspondent being unreasonably critical of the author.

Objective findings

Irritability is revealed by cursing or critical comments. The voice may be raised, the eyes wide or rolled and there may be sighing and hissing. (Figure 11) Alternatively, there may be refusal to speak or enter into conversation. There may be a tendency to break things and in the extreme, to physical assault.

More commonly the irritable patient simply looks tense and is easily startled and annoyed.

The presence of irritability suggests a range of psychiatric disorders including mania, depression, paranoid psychosis and attention deficit disorder. Also exclude stimulant use, drug withdrawal, delirium of other causes and common irritable, difficult personality.

Anxiety

Subjective experience

Anxious patients describe feeling 'churned up', 'worried', 'frightened' and 'up set'. They may suffer 'butterflies'.

Objective findings

The anxious patient is often pale, looking frightened and restless. The hands are often sweating and tremulous, clenched or touching the face or hair and straightening the clothes. There may be much clearing of the throat and difficulty with articulation due to dryness of the mouth. There may be frequent micturition.

One view of agitated depression is that this is co-existence of anxiety and depression. It is my view that irritability is less frequent in uncomplicated anxiety than in agitated depression.

The symptom of anxiety is present in the various anxiety disorders, depressive disorders, schizophrenia and drug withdrawal. Being interviewed about emotional matters may produce some anxiety in some people.

4. Affect

Affect is another term about which there is some difference of opinion. This discontent has roots in the similarities between affect and mood and past failure to agree on universal definitions. An example of the disarray in the area is that until recently, the mood disorders were called 'affective disorders'. The DSM-III-R was the first to use the term mood disorder and the IDC-10 now employs what is apparently transitional terminology, 'Mood [Affective] Disorders'. It may have been better to discard the old and recruit new terms, but this approach has been resisted and there has been an attempt to draft new definitions for the old terms.

To set the scene, be aware that emotion has been described as a complex feeling state with psychic, somatic and behavioural components. It is generally reactive to external events and such changes are mostly immediate – the moment the quizmaster says 'Yes! You have won $1000 000!', the contestant is happy, tachycardic and smiling. (We do not need to bother with whether the smile came before the feeling of happiness or the other way around, as long as we can agree that the feeling followed the environmental stimulus reasonably closely.)

Affect is now described (Kaplan and Saddock, 1991) as: 1) the expression of emotion as observed by others; and 2) varying over time, in response to changing emotional states. The first part of this description is interchangeable with the fourth part of the definition of mood, that is, evidence of the emotion which is observable by others. The second part of this description, that affect will change in response to changing emotional states, is distinct from the definition of mood, in which the emotion is stated to be 'sustained'.

(Other descriptions of affect include: 1) the external manifestation of an internal feeling state; and 2) what the observer observes when an individual is experiencing an emotion. Thus, there is agreement that affect is a signal.)

In a recent edition of the DSM it was stated that affect is to mood what weather is to climate. Thus, the more changeable nature of affect as compared to mood was emphasised.

In the interview situation, subtle changes in affect (the response signal) are expected with changes in stimulus, that is, with changes in topic. This means different affects and variations in the depth of particular affects (changes in quality and quantity of affect). Many of the observations that contribute to the evaluation of affect are mentioned elsewhere in the mental state examination. The observations on which an assessment of affect is based include: the voice, mentioned under 'Talk' – whether there are changes is tone or volume; the ability to smile appropriately; movements – whether there are hand or body movements; whether the patient displays any interpersonal warmth or has any interest; energy or motivation toward any goal; and whether there is evidence of the range of feelings including love, hate, anger, regret, hope, expectation and empathy.

A consideration of mood and affect in depression and schizophrenia illustrates some points. Depression is a mood disorder – mood is a sustained emotional state. The face of the depressed patient is usually immobile – an objective findings with respect to the mood – an immobile face is also an objective finding with respect to affect. Affect changes with the emotions, but if the emotion is sustained, there will be little change of the affect. Thus, in depression, the emotional experience is depression, the objective findings are of depression and the affect is accordingly remarkable (perhaps flat – see later for details). It is of interest that mood disorders resolve or respond and as this happens the affect returns to normal, that is, it begins to vary over time and with the changes of topic of conversation.

Schizophrenia is a disorder in which there is loss of the emotions. Because of the loss of emotional life, patients with schizophrenia tend to have immobile faces. They usually do not complain of feeling depressed. When pressed they often report having no feelings. (Figure 12). As there is a reduction in emotional life there is little change in affect over time. Schizophrenia does not resolve or respond as depression does, therefore, the individual does not regain emotion and affect does not return as it may in depression.

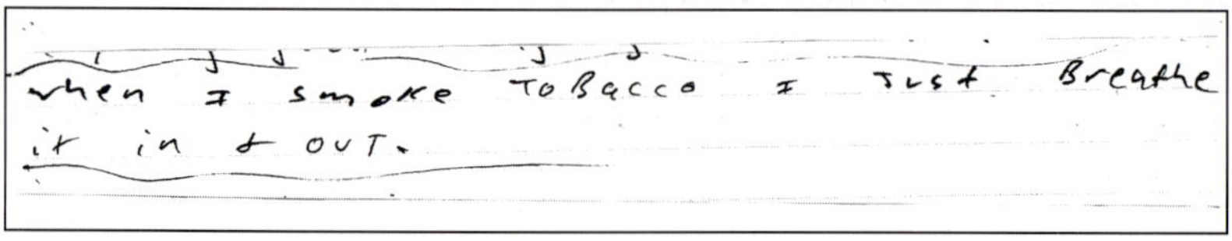

Figure 12. This patient suffered schizophrenia. Here he was expressing the subjective experience of loss of affect, which was objectively manifest as flat affect. Research shows that many people with schizophrenia smoke because the effect of nicotine is pleasurable. This man, however, was adamant that smoking no longer gave him any pleasure whatsoever – "I just breathe in & out".

Thus, the emotional experience differs in depression and schizophrenia, but the affect may have similarities.

Humour appreciation has a characteristic objective component or affect. Shammi and Stuss (1999) recently provided information on humour appreciation – a defining human attribute. To place their observations in context, the appreciation of humour calls for the ability to: 1) perceive; 2) detect surprise (incongruity) in a punch-line; 3) resolve that incongruity by establishing a coherence between different parts of the joke; 4) interpret information in the light of past personal experiences; and 5) integrate cognitive and emotional information.

Precise pathophysiology of the various affects is scarce. Shammi and Stuss (1999) looked at localised brain damage and found 'only patients with right frontal lobe damage displayed significantly muted physical-emotional responsiveness to the humorous stimuli...'. They postulate that right frontal lobe damage results in disruption of integration of cognitive and emotional information. The corollary is that the right frontal lobe plays an important part in humour appreciation and the associated affect.

Affect is assessed during the entire examination process. Attention is paid to the range and depth of affect when discussing the presenting complaint, the relationship with family members (including those deceased), the children (or the lack of children), achievements and other events from the personal history. It is expected that these topics will trigger different emotions and that there will be different affective signals. Consideration is also given to the affect aroused by patient–interviewer interactions. A joke may be attempted. If a depressed patient responds to any stimuli with a smile or evidence of happiness, this congruent affect may be alternatively reported as 'reactive mood'.

A large range of labels and descriptions has evolved for the classification of affect. Too many categories reduce reliability. The following trim list is recommended.

Appropriate (normal) affect

The affect suggests the full range and depth of internal feeling states which is culturally consistent with the conversation (which introduces various subjects) or interaction.

Flat affect

When the affect is flat, there is little if any change in the quality and quantity of affect with the introduction of different topics of conversation.

Restricted and blunted affect are terms which have, in the past, been used as alternatives to flat affect, however, Kaplan and Saddock (1991) have arranged the three in order of degree. I recommend using only one term, flat affect. The first task is to determine whether flat affect is present or not, and if it is, a comment on whether it is mild, moderate or severe may be attempted. The point has been made above that the affect in schizophrenia and depression may appear similar (although arising by different processes). Where there are few hand gestures, the voice monotonous and the face immobile, it is correct to use the term, flat affect. There is a tendency to use the term 'depressed' affect. This is not recommended, as it presupposes the diagnosis. It is errant to use the term 'depressed' affect in the description of schizophrenia.

Flat affect or similar observations may be encountered in Parkinson's disease (idiopathic and drug induced), hypothyroidism and other neurological conditions (e.g., dystrophia myotonica) in addition to the already mentioned conditions, schizophrenia and depression.

Inappropriate (incongruent) affect

Inappropriate or incongruent affect indicates an internal feeling state which is not culturally consistent with the conversation or interaction. Theoretically, this term could be applied where there is flat affect, but the term inappropriate affect is usually reserved for more curious situations such as inappropriate mirth or anger. The word 'inappropriate' means that the affect is inappropriate to the thought content. The most obvious example is when a patient is discussing a sad event, but displays apparent pleasure (laughter while discussing being sacked or the death of a loved person).

This category must be used with caution. Laughter may arise from arousal. An anxious individual who is embarrassed by a certain event (spilling coffee at an important meeting) or topic of their history may defend with a laugh. The emotional pain of loss may be shrugged off with a laugh.

Further, it is necessary to have access to the content of thought before it is possible to comment on whether or not the affect is inappropriate. For example, if an individual has a long and deep dislike for a parent, laughter at the mention of their death may be appropriate rather than inappropriate. Inability to get access to the content of thought of psychotic individuals makes use of this term problematic.

Inappropriate or incongruous affect is observed in disorganised (hebephrenic) schizophrenia. Here it may be termed 'fatuous' affect. There may be giggling and failure to respond affectively or behaviourally to serious situations – such patients may be described as demonstrating 'silliness' and 'shallowness'. Rather than create an additional category, fatuous affect may be included under the present heading. (Figure 13)

Rarely, patients with other forms of schizophrenia may become suddenly and unnecessarily violent. Subsequently, in discussions, such patients may show lack of remorse or distress when faced with the consequences of their actions. Appearing unconcerned, in such circumstances, may be described in terms of inappropriate affect.

The individual with antisocial personality will display a callous disregard for the consequences of action, as may the individual with mental retardation. Apparent inappropriate affect may occur during states of very high arousal.

Instead I fumbled along, failing miserably in an under-staffed bank, with double the work load that I could do in one day. I was sacked. Most of the time I was in a daze and I never knew if I had served any customers accurately or not, anyway after I got my notice I was working in a Commonwealth sub-branch in Highton. For the day I was $50 out, earlier at Corio Village I was $500 short in the balancing of the money at the end of the day. I got determined as we were on our way to the bank headquarters, I made up my mind that I was going to do better. As I was deciding this for a while, getting more and more determined suddenly Heaven opened and I looked up and felt and heard God laugh. It was a happy, benevolent, empathetic laughter that immediately made me feel better. I saw the laughter stream down from Heaven to me. The last thing on earth I wanted to do was laugh. I was so, so serious and I was a bit annoyed that God didn't share my concern. Perhaps He knew something that I didn't. Anyway getting out of the car I saw Brian Ferbisher, my best friend from church. He was sitting down in the gutter underneath a sign (I think it was a bus stop). Well, when he saw me, Brian stood up and was walking across the footpath staring at me with a big smile and laughter in his eye. I said hello and looked at him staring at me until I was about ten yards past him. I think it was the most evenly contested staring match seen in Bendigo that year.

Figure 13. This was from by the same young man who wrote Figure 6.

He describes himself as having been 'in a daze' and being unsure of whether he had performed his duties properly. Rather than having a problem with conscious level as the word 'daze' might suggest, the writer is probably describing the subjective difficulty of performing exacting duties while disabled by formal thought disorder and distracted by other psychotic experiences.

He describes seeing God's laugh 'stream down from heaven'. This was an hallucinatory, psychotic experience which is difficult to classify.

The last sentence, 'I think it was the most evenly contested staring match seen in Bendigo that year' may appear to be a clever piece of humorous writing. The alternative and probably correct interpretation is that it represents mild formal thought disorder and inappropriate/fatuous affect characteristic of disorganised (hebephrenic) schizophrenia.

Labile affect

The affect changes suddenly and frequently, suggesting sudden and frequent changes in emotions, but these changes are culturally excessive in the given environment.

It is important to identify labile affect and to differentiate it from inappropriate affect. In labile affect there are frequent shifts of affect, often from one extreme to the other. This may occur in response to a minimal stimulus. Thus, a patient may respond to mention of a distant moderately unhappy event with tears and great distress, and subsequently be moved by an encouraging remark to hilarity and happyness. Left alone, such a patient may display a range of affects, presumably associated with spontaneous thoughts and consequent emotions. Labile affect (reflecting labile emotions) is commonly described as being subjectively unpleasant.

As with inappropriate affect, labile affect may result in sudden, unnecessary violence.

Labile affect may be observed in the aftermath of severe psychological trauma, intoxication, substance withdrawal, dementia, hypoxia and other causes of delirium as well as schizophrenia, attention deficit disorder and mixed mood disorder (symptoms of mania and depression occurring simultaneously).

5. Thought

The assessment of thought is difficult. It calls for knowledge and experience. Like craniotomy, it is a technical skill. While other health and social services workers (police, clergy, surgeons) can give a fair account of some aspects of the mental state of a patient, it is only with special training that thought can be assessed. Abnormalities in thought are powerful diagnostic pointers. Thus, skill in the assessment of thought is an essential part of the armamentarium of clinicians working in psychiatry.

Throughout the mental state examination, the patient is thinking – without thinking the patient cannot, for example, give answers to the memory test. However, traditionally, only two aspects of thinking are covered by this heading: form (the connections between bits of information) and content. This division will be used here, but under form will be included flight of ideas and poverty of thought, both of which may be problems of rate rather than connection.

Thought is largely assessed by the examination of speech. To the extent that speech may not precisely reflect thought, care must be taken to avoid assumptions.

Thought is also reflected in behaviour. A person who places a sign on his front door warning that aliens have landed and barricades himself inside the house armed with various weapons, would appear to be suffering from a disorder of the content of thought. Behaviour gives less clear evidence of disorder of the form of thought, for although poor quality thinking leads to poor quality planning and ultimately, poor behavioural outcome (such as in failure to secure employment), behaviour also depends on a range of additional factors including personality, motivation and cognition.

On occasions, behaviour may predict with considerable certainty, disorder of the form of thought. A carpenter was admitted to hospital with disorder of the form of thought and disorganised behaviour. In the Occupational Therapy Department he set about making a cross (Christian) to hang on the wall of his home. Rather than fix together two pieces of wood symmetrically and at right angles, he nailed two pieces of wood together such that the left and right arms were different lengths, and the angles they made with the upright were not right angles. Apparently to correct the asymmetry, additional pieces of wood were roughly nailed to the arms. These increased the weight and made the central join unstable. Perhaps to increase stability, he then nailed pieces of wood between the ends of cross, thus converting it into a square with a cross in the middle. The patient's parents were worried by the quality of this structure and stated that it was much below his usual standard. When the patient recovered he was embarrassed by his cross and could not explain his poor workmanship.

For clinicians to make useful decisions about the presence or absence of disorders of thought, they must have clear definitions and a small number of categories from which to choose. The larger the number of categories, the lower the reliability, and it is a pity to waste these valuable pointers.

This field becomes more complicated with every author who proposes a change or addition. Berrios (1996) states 'After the First World War, papers carrying the words 'language' or 'thought' disorder in schizophrenia began to appear: in the 1930s the trickle had become a flood...'

I propose using established definitions, but leaving out some categories (such as 'knight's move thinking' and 'condensation') to reduce the number of choices. The examiner needs to learn less than a dozen types of disorder of the form thought to master the area. It may be useful to know of other definitions for theoretical reasons, but they will not be needed in clinical practice.

Form

Form means the 'arrangement of parts' (Oxford Dictionary). Disturbances in the form of thought are disturbances in the logical process of thought – put more simply, disturbances in the logical connections between ideas.

Clinicians may need to be vigilant to detect disorders of the form of thought (a slightly shorter synonym being, 'formal thought disorders').

In everyday life we pay attention to the content of our conversations with friends and colleagues, paying particular attention to the content of 'the bottom line'. We tend to filter out the 'noise' of changes of subject and direction. As, in the mental state examination we need to assess the form of thought specifically, the examiner is encouraged to spend time studying the form of thought in everyday conversations to become familiar with the 'normal range'.

The form of thought is assessed throughout the initial interview and at all subsequent contacts. If the interview is a highly structured series of questions and answers, disorder of the form of thought will be less apparent. Accordingly, the examiner may arrange opportunities for the form of thought to be revealed – this means periods with little structure, when patients are encouraged to speak freely and required to impose their own structure.

Thought processes can also be tested through the use of abstract questions. Such questions give few clues on how to structure answers and there is, therefore, greater chance of loss of logical process/connections. Religious or philosophical questions are useful, and should be tailored to suit the patient – if patients have talked about having faith, it is reasonable to ask, 'Why do you believe in God?'. If patients have talked about outer space or scientific theories, it is reasonable to ask, 'How could time travel contribute to pollution?' or, 'What would the relationship be between the space creatures you have described and the Christian God?'

Other tasks with abstract material include giving explanations of the meaning of proverbs, such as, 'A stitch in time', 'People who live in glass houses' and 'Still waters run deep'. It is imperative, of course, to give proper consideration to the intelligence, education and cultural background of people when assessing their response to abstract questions. For example, those with relatively low intelligence and little education are likely to give concrete answers, which might otherwise represent formal thought disorder. Thus, when in doubt, abstract questions are avoided, and the form of thought is judged using only the conversation that occurs during the interview.

An excellent example is given by Solovay *et al.*, (1986)

Interviewer, 'Why should we pay taxes?'.

Patient, 'Taxation, we have representation... taxation without representation is treason...'.

Here, the loss of logical connections between ideas is clear, so there is disorder of the form of thought. Treason is usually clandestine and damaging, it is the sort of issue that worries patients who have paranoid delusions. Thus, the mention of treason in an ordinary doctor–patient discussion suggest that the patient may also have a disorder of content of thought.

At times, when thought disorder is suspected, the clinician may sit in silence with the patient for a short time. Silence is uncommon in everyday conversation and the patient may find the experience anxiety provoking. Anxiety can accentuate disorders of thought (in those with mental disorders and those without). The silence offers no structure or cue for comment. Accordingly, a patient may break a silence with a thought-disordered statement. Avoid this procedure if the patient appears to find such silences distressing.

Finally, for diagnostic and progress assessment purposes, it is essential to record verbatim examples of formal thought disorder in the patient's file. While dramatic or humorous thought disorder may be remembered for a few minutes, the more common, less remarkable examples, which carry the same diagnostic power, are very difficult to remember. This is partly because of the lack of logical connections (we all need order for optimal mentation), and partly because when formal thought disorder is present it is necessary to listen very closely and this makes the keeping of mental notes most difficult. It is recommended that the observer write down verbatim extracts as the patient speaks, either directly into the file, or on other paper from which they can be transcribed later.

Derailment

Derailment occurs when a train jumps off the track. Kaplan and Saddock (1991) define derailment as gradual or sudden deviation in the train of thought. Andreasen (1979) defines derailment as 'A pattern of ... speech in which the ideas slip off the track onto another one which is clearly but obliquely related, or onto one which is completely unrelated'. (Figures 13, 14, 15, 16).

The term derailment was introduced to replace the earlier term, 'loosening of associations' (which had been introduced by Eugene Bleuler in 1911 – he thought that looseness of associations represented the fundamental disturbance in schizophrenia – he also introduced the term schizophrenia). It was said that loosening of associations had been used indiscriminately and had thereby lost meaning.

In an example of the lack of clarity in the field, Kaplan and Saddock (1991) state that 'derailment is sometimes used synonymously with loosening of associations' but then go on to give separate definitions (between

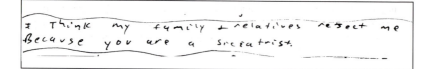

Figure 14. This was written by a young man who suffered schizophrenia. There was no evidence that his family and relatives rejected him. This was a disorder of content.

'Because you are a siciatrist' was not a feature of disordered content, rather it was a feature of disordered form of thought. The patient had the view that his family rejected him because he suffered mental illness. In the above example the patient derailed from the fact that he had a mental illness onto the track that he was being treated by a psychiatrist.

It is when the brain has recovered from coition, and when it is fed by pure fruit blood so to speak, that one feels a Divine content. When the brain receives the perversion of shocks of our forcible coition, that injures it in the first place; then a hot meat diet clogs the body with waste nitrogenous matter, and that tells on the feelings, on the tone and joy of life. Then alcohol is put directly into the stomach perhaps, still more lowering tone, joy and love. All the affections are perverted, hate is born (hate has a purely subjective origin), and things, one should think, are just about as bad and "degenerate" as possible. Not so: tobacco or opium are now resorted to, to try to, remedy this restless misery. Then perhaps this coition-injured, meat and alcohol poisoned, nicotine solution of a man is called upon to give his decision on some vital question, such as a declaration of war, or of the best way to treat the "criminal", the poor, outcast, widow or orphan.

Our pathetic reliance on amusements, fiction, theatres and "pastimes" is not the least evidence in proof of our injury.

Because a man has a rush of blood to his head, or any other part of his body, that does not prove it to be a natural function.

Every married man and woman has distorted and "knitted" eyebrows.

The best way to meet the difficulty will be candid discussion between the sexes. Candour alone will clear away half our troubles, and render us more sane on the subject. Children should be ...

Figure 15. This extract is from "The Answer" a pamphlet written by William James Chidley (1860-1916). He was a photographer and artist for much of his life. In the last years of his life, however, he traveled extensively and lectured in streets and parks. He spoke against 'unnatural coition' and in favor of 'natural coition', nudity and a diet of fruit and nuts.

He was arrested many times for disturbing the peace and similar offenses. He was declared insane and placed in different psychiatric hospitals at different times. He died in Callen Park psychiatric hospital.

This type of behaviour, lecturing in the streets on religious and moral issues, is fairly uncommon today. It was, perhaps, more common in the past and the term 'religious mania' was applied. While many of these people may have suffered mania, it is also probable that others suffered what would now be termed schizophrenia or delusional disorder – both of which may manifest erotic and grandiose delusions.

In the extract, the reader is impressed by the fervor of the writer, but it is difficult to follow the specifics of his argument. There are many suggestions of derailment, a good example being the statement, 'Every married man and woman has distorted and "knitted" eyebrows' – which is obliquely, at best, related to the previous idea.

which students cannot discriminate). Thus, the terms can be used interchangeably, but only one (any authoritative) definition need be learned.

Derailment is rarely complained of by the patient and is easily dismissed by the doctor as a mere eccentricity of expression – but it may be an ominous indicator of a devastating disorder. (Figure 14, 15). To appre-

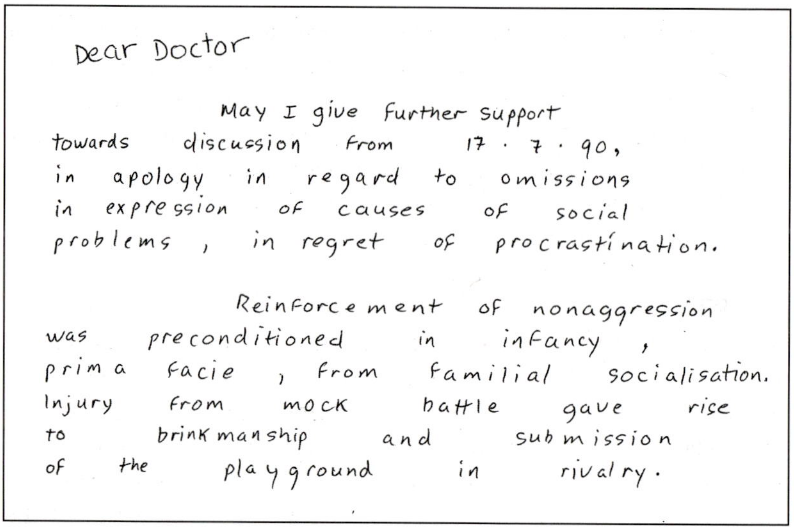

Dear Doctor

        May I give further support towards discussion from 17 . 7 . 90, in apology in regard to omissions in expression of causes of social problems , in regret of procrastination.

        Reinforcement of nonaggression was preconditioned in infancy , prima facie , from familial socialisation. Injury from mock battle gave rise to brinkmanship and submission of the playground in rivalry.

Figure 16. This is the first two paragraphs of a three page letter from a patient to his psychiatrist. The patient suffered Obsessive–Compulsive Personality Disorder (OCPD) and had been in supportive therapy for one year.

At a recent session the psychiatrist made what he considered to be a benign comment about the patient's tendency to procrastinate. The letter was written because the patient did not want to disappoint the psychiatrist and was apologetic about his slow progress.

Characteristic of OCPD, there is little spontaneity or warmth. The patient has focused so much energy on accurately expressing his thoughts that his style has become stilted. However, thought processes which remain on track should not be mistaken for derailment.

ciate the potential importance of derailment, an analogy is drawn with physical medicine. In derailment, the patient is following a train of thought and suddenly veers off onto a different track. If, during a neurological examination, the same patient was asked to walk across the room toward the examiner, and half way across he/she suddenly turned off at a 45 degree angle and walked into a wall, the examiner would be concerned. Which is more important, walking or thinking? This is not a serious question; it is used to emphasise the potential importance of derailment. Among the most disabling consequences of schizophrenia is the inability to budget, plan and carry out activities. I believe that thought disorder lies at the root of these problems.

Derailment is one of a number of types of formal thought disorder. However, it is my opinion that derailment is a basic type and that at least some of the other types of formal thought disorder are simply elaborations of derailment.

Tangentiality was once equivalent to derailment, but was redefined by Andreasen (1979) to apply only to answers and not to spontaneous speech. This term can be applied when a question is asked and the patient gives an answer which has 'slipped off the track' and is either obliquely or even unrelated to the question. In clinical practice, to simplify our task, it is recommended that the distinction between derailment and tangentiality be ignored and that we use the term derailment for both.

An example from my recent experience:

Interviewer, 'How old are you?'

Patient, 'I feel young sometimes'.

With respect to the above example, at first glance it might appear that I am making a mountain out of a mole hill, as this is the sort of response we all might make, sliding off the question but communicating other important information. After all, in this anti-discrimination era people are encouraged to assert that they are '55 (or any number) years young' rather than 55 years 'old'. But this came fairly early in an interview, in which demographic data was being collected. That is, in a part of the interview where there is structure and the conventional response is to provide a factual rather than a philosophical response. In this setting, such a response suggests, but does not prove, disorder of the form of thought.

[On the topic of tangentiality, Kaplan and Saddock (1991) give the definition of 'inability to have goal-directed associations of thought' – a good example of how thought disorder can become unnecessarily complicated.]

As mentioned a couple of times, isolated examples of derailment may occur in the conversation of normal individuals. Where there are more frequent examples it is necessary to exclude the dysphasias (of vascular, traumatic, degenerative or other organic origin). Derailment may occur in mania (see later, under flight of ideas) and depression. It is characteristically found in schizophrenia, particularly in subtypes with younger onset. Derailment will also be found in schizophreniform disorder and schizotypal personality disorder.

Flight of ideas (includes clanging)

In flight of ideas rapid, continuous verbalisations are associated with constant shifting from one idea to another. (Figures 17 to 20).

Wing *et al.* (1974) describe three types: 1) where there is rhyming, alliteration or clanging, e.g., ill, illegitimate, illusion; 2) where there is an association by meaning, including opposites, e.g., white, black, coffin; and 3) where there is distraction, e.g., a patient talking about his appetite sees another patient walk past the window, assumes that patient is going for ECT and starts talking about ECT.

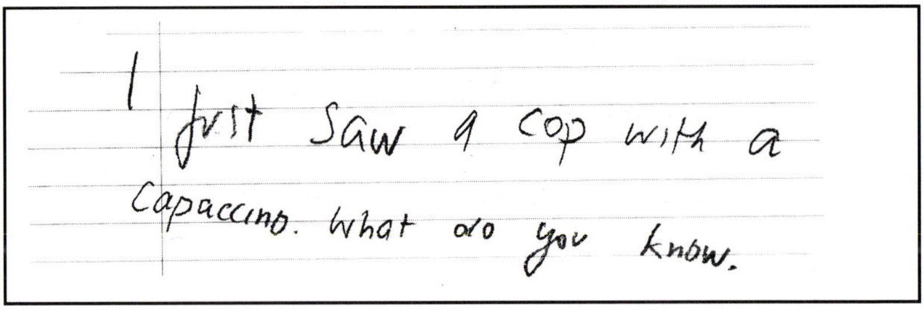

> I just saw a cop with a Capaccino. What do you know.

Figure 17. This was written by a young man who was suffering acute mania. He was overactive. He would leave the hospital and go walking in the city. On his return he would leave messages at my office.

Sighting a policeman drinking coffee is an trivial event and would not usually be considered worthy of reporting. That he did so suggests pressure of speech (he was pressured to keep speaking/ writing).

It is also interesting that in these two short lines there are examples of two forms of clanging. The syllables 'cop' and 'cap' constitute and alliteration. The words at the ends of these sentences 'capaccino' and 'know' rhyme. The sentence 'What do you know' adds no new information and is largely a vehicle for the rhyme.

I believe that the difference between types two and three above is simply the site of the distraction and that they are both examples of flight of ideas in which there is movement from one topic to another via an association of meanings. In type two the distraction occurs internally and in type three the distraction occurs externally to the patient. But such debate (like a wrangle which went on about the difference between knight's move thinking and looseness of associations) is sterile from a clinical perspective and can be ignored by the clinician – given present knowledge.

It is of interest that the example of clanging given above 'ill, illegitimate, illusion' is not a rhyme, but alliteration. Rhyme is 'agreement in the terminal sounds of lines of words', while alliteration is 'the same consonant sound at the commencement of two or more stressed syllables of a word group'. Thus, clanging may include rhyme and alliteration.

Dealing with clanging, Andreasen has also drawn attention to punning. In an early draft of her Thought, Language and Communication Scale, she gave the example, 'I'm not trying to make noise ... I'm not trying to make sense (cents) anymore. I'm trying to make dollars'. Here the sound of the word 'sense' brings in a new topic, which is the essence of punning. In flight of ideas, punning does not need to be placed in a category distinct from rhyme. Not surprisingly, with high mood elevation the punning of flight of ideas can be frequent, amusing and apparently clever.

Many of the debates about the mental state of particular patients centre on whether what they manifest is derailment or flight of ideas. The

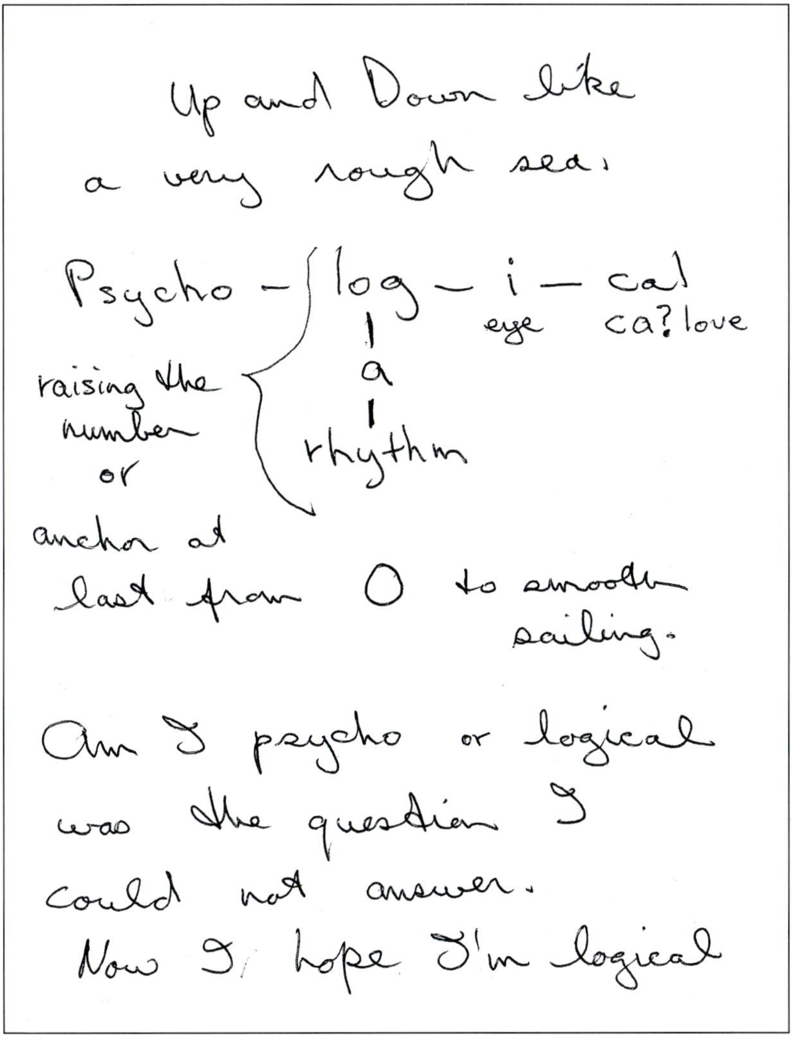

Up and Down like
a very rough sea.

Psycho — log — i — cal
eye   ca? love
raising the
number   a
or   rhythm

anchor at
last from O to smooth
sailing.

Am I psycho or logical
was the question I
could not answer.
Now I hope I'm logical

Figure 18. This was written/composed by a young person who was suffering from mania. The association of psychological and logarithm is an example of clanging.

A central feature is the word 'psychological'. A possible explanation is as follows. The letters 'log' reminded her of the word 'logarithm' which is written vertically. The word 'logarithm' suggested 'raising the number', which then suggested raising an 'anchor'. This brought to mind the idea of 'smooth sailing', which may have suggested the idea which she added at the top of the page, 'up and down like a very rough sea'. The 'up and down' is probably also suggested by the raising of the anchor and the up and down cycling of her bipolar disorder.

Finally, she added the words 'Am I psycho or logical'. At the time of writing, in popular parlance, the world 'psycho' meant mentally ill. She finished with 'Now I hope I'm logical'. These bottom lines suggest a sense of fun which is a common accompaniment of the mood elevation of mania. In the last sentence the patient writes that she hopes she is 'logical' – this may indicate that she is aware that she has been illogical (or psychotic) in the past and that at the current time she had a degree of insight.

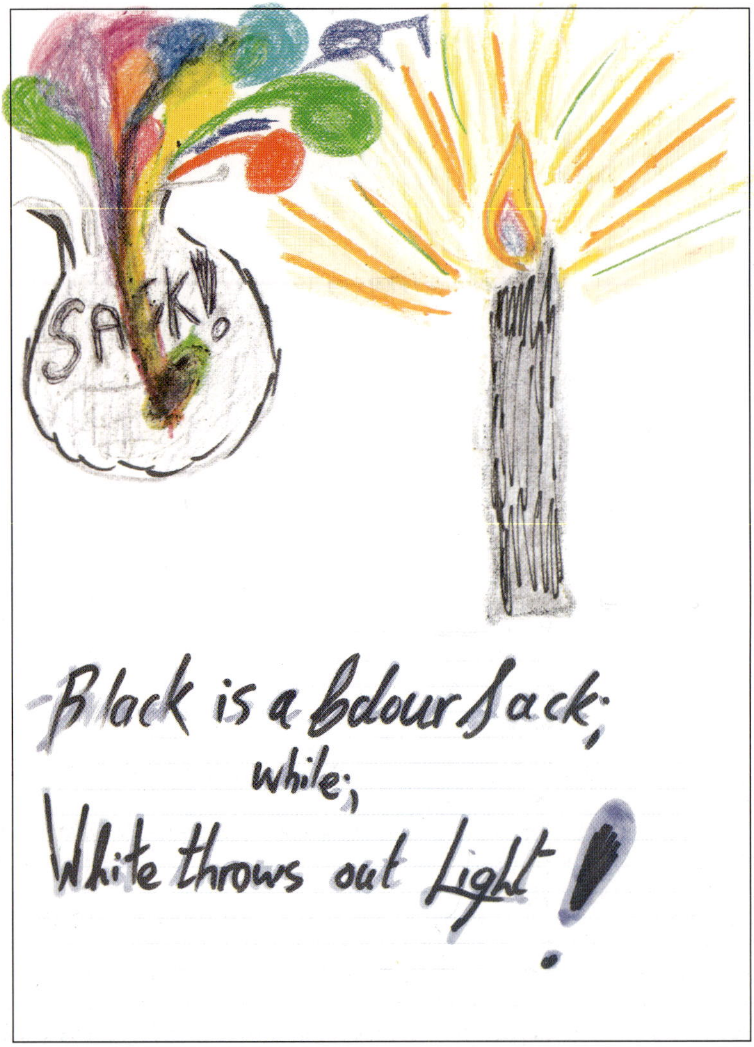

Figure 19. This composition was made by a young science graduate during an episode of mania.

A number of features suggest mania. First, the drawings are colorful and hurried. Second, they are in crayon and lack sophistication. Thirdly, 'black' and 'sack', and 'white' and 'light', while perhaps masquerading as the rhyme of poetry, are clanging associations. Finally, the information is poorly communicated. It can be argued that white reflects or throws 'back' all light; to state that it throws 'out' light suggests a process akin to radioactivity and is misleading.

The reader may disagree on this last point and have the view that the patient is being creative and I, pedestrian. It is the case that people with mania, via rapid thinking, can have new and even brilliant ideas. Unfortunately, because of this rapidity of thinking or for some other reason, the ideas of the person with mania are often not subjected to critical evaluation. The above illustration comes from a book of writings, some of which, if not this particular piece, lack the clarity of thought and communication skills expected of a science graduate.

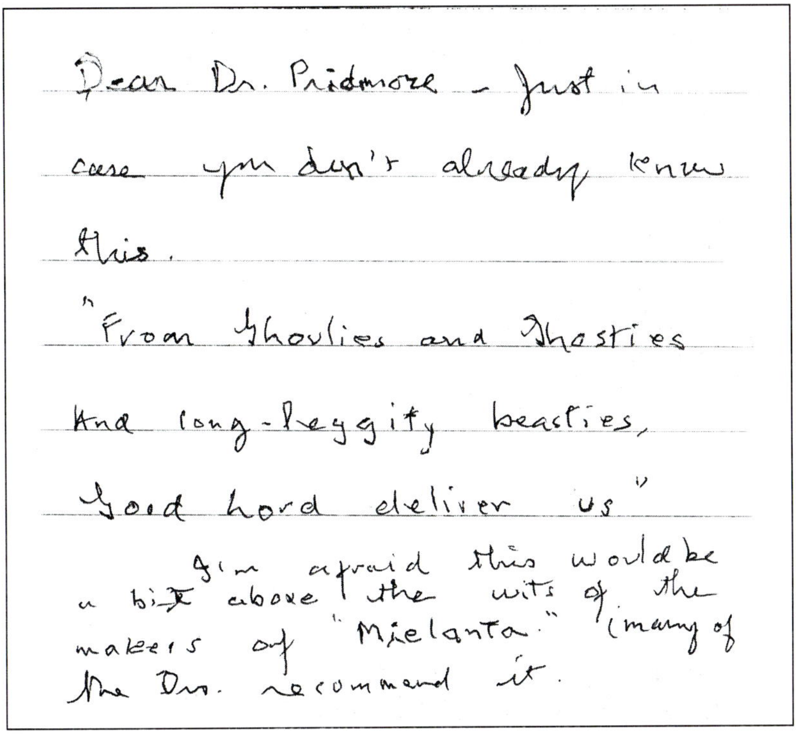

Dear Dr. Pridmore – Just in case you don't already know this.

"From Ghoulies and Ghosties And long-leggity beasties, Good Lord deliver us"

I'm afraid this would be a bit above the wits of the makers of "Mielanta" (many of the Drs. recommend it.

Figure 20. This is a further example from the elderly lady mentioned in Figure 1. It was written some years later during a subsequent manic episode.

This letter is not quite as remarkable as it may first appear, as the passage 'From Ghoulies and Ghosties and long-leggity beasties, Good Lord deliver us' is, in fact, an ancient prayer from the Cornwall region of Great Britain.

It is not clear why the patient thought this prayer would be of interest to her doctor. After the prayer comes the mention of the wits of the makers of 'Mielanta' (apparently a misspelling of the proprietary name Mylanta, an antacid). It is difficult to find a connection between the prayer and Mylanta. The reason for communicating the information that many doctors recommend Mylanta is unclear. There is a disorder of the form of thought and because there was pressure of speech it is best termed flight of ideas.

old view was that there is something different in the quality of the connections which justifies the use of separate categories – in one category connections between the dislocated ideas were believed to be more understandable than in the other. This view had scientific weaknesses and no good operational differences have been found. Andreasen (1979) states 'flight of ideas is a derailment that occurs rapidly in the context of pressured speech'.

My recommendation is that the Andreasen view be endorsed, that in the absence of pressure of speech the term derailment be applied and in

MEDICAL RESEARCH.

EXAMINATION OF HEAD.

(1) PROFESSIONAL (2) NON-PROFESSIONAL.

EFFECT OF POLISHING OF SHOES OVER THE TIME BETWEEN THIS POLISH AND THE NEXT POLISH.
UNCONSCIOUS OBSERVATIONS AND AFFECT UPON HEAD OVER THE LIFE SPAN OF A HUMAN BEING. — SERVICE BOOTS AND CIVILIAN SHOES.

A BIOLOGY STUDY OF GARDENING AND FARMING FRATERNITIES - EFFECT OF PROCESS OF BUILDING UP SOIL AND HUMUS IN THE SOIL — VARIOUS TYPES OF SOIL. — SEA AND GEOLOGY STUDIES.

THE PROCESS OF DRY-FIREWOOD UPON HEAD (CUTTING.) AND A RELATIONSHIP

a

MEDICINE
FANG AFTER FANG CLEANED A

NUCLEAR PHYSICS —
WHERE DANGER EXISTS OF HUMAN-BEINGS BECOMING MORALLY UNSAFE DUE TO INSUFFICIENT SCIENTIFIC TRAINING, IT IS THE USUAL PRACTICE TO CONSIDER A PERSON DEAD BUT NOT ALIVE UNDER CIRCUMSTANCES WHERE HIS THOUGHT AND IDEAS ARE SUBJECTED TO INTENSE INTERROGATION BY SECTIONS OF A POPULATION UNDER CONDITIONS OF NUCLEAR-RESEARCH.
INDEED HE WOULD BE A DANGER TO HIMSELF, HIS FAMILY, HIS FELLOW EMPLOYEES AND HIS COMMUNITY, IF HE WERE TORMENTED WITH UNPRODUCTIVE AND IMMORAL HUMAN-BEINGS WHO HAD NOT BEEN SUFFICIENTLY TRAINED TO TAKE RESPONSIBILITY IN RAISING LEVELS OF HUMAN-ENDEAVOUR. THEY WOULD BE MENACE TO THEM-SELVES AND EVERYONE ABOUT THEM SHOULD THEY UNSOBER, AND WERE SUBJECTED TO PARTICULAR TORMENTS OF NUCLEAR RESEARCH.
DID HE RECOVER IN A SECOND.?

b

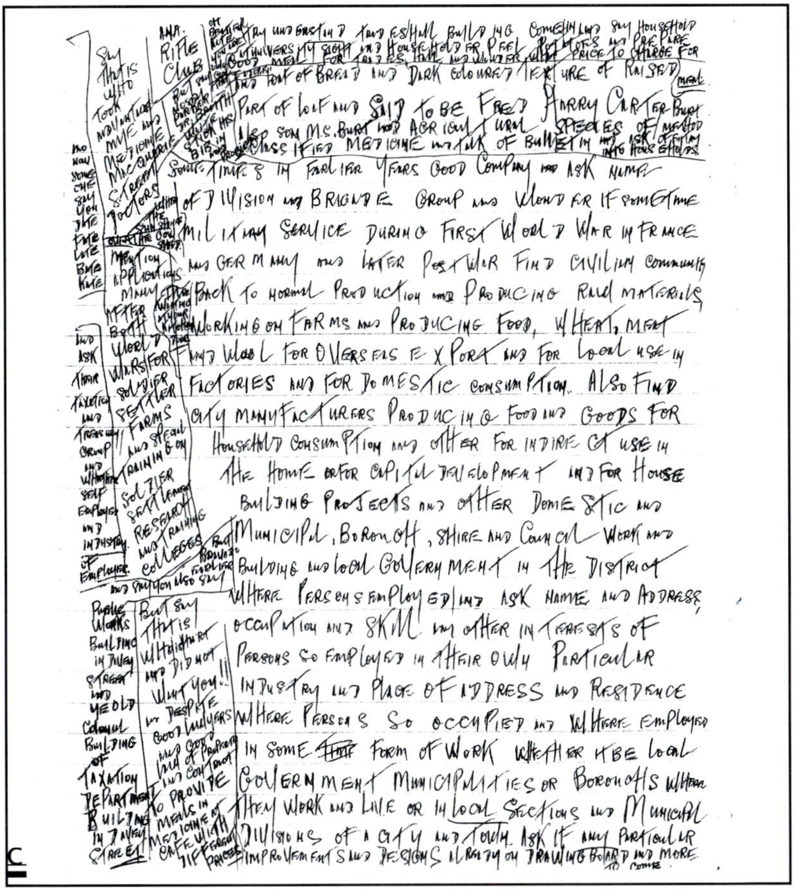

Figure 21a, b, c. These three examples were written by a man who trained in mathematics at university during the Second World War.

After graduating he worked in an administrative post for more than a decade before developing schizophrenia. He then spent some years in a psychiatric hospital.

While in hospital he wrote over 600 pages of his thoughts in five exercise books. In each book his writing was presented slightly differently. In one book (a) the printing is clear and well spaced, in another (b) the printing is widely spaced with the majority of the words underlined, and in another book (c) the printing is very cramped with two or more columns packed in the margin and at the top and bottom of each page.

Two of the books were of poor quality paper and as the patient used a fountain pen, the writing is illegible. In the three remaining books the printing is legible, but it is impossible to derive meaning. For instance, in the first example on page one is the heading 'MEDICAL RESEARCH, EXAMINATION OF THE HEAD'. The first line of text, however, deals with the polishing of shoes. The influence of his education can be detected in the entry 'EFFECTS OF POLISHING OF SHOES OVER THE TIME BETWEEN THE POLISH AND THE NEXT POLISH', which is reminiscent of the approach to a scientific question.

It is possible to determine examples of derailment but much of what appears in these pages is incoherent thought disorder.

the presence of pressure of speech the term flight of ideas be applied. The argument then becomes not between derailment and flight, but between the presence or absence of pressure – a question on which agreement is easier to achieve. With pressure of speech there is an increase in speed of talk, the voice is usually loud and the patient is difficult to interrupt (this is dealt with in more detail under Talk).

Flight of ideas most often occurs in mania, however it also occurs in schizophrenia. Intoxication with stimulants must be excluded. I have also seen a small number of cases of infarction of the cerebellum in which the patient was loud, disinhibited and manifesting what could pass as flight of ideas.

Incoherence

Incoherent thought is incomprehensible due to extreme loss of logical connections, distortion of grammar and idiosyncratic use of words (Figure 21, 22).

The following example is from Andreasen (1979).

Interviewer: 'What do you think about current political issues like the energy crisis?'

Patient: 'They're destroying too many cattle and oil just to make soap. If we need soap when you can jump into a pool of water, and then when you go to buy your gasoline, my folks always thought they should get pop, but the best thing to get is motor oil, and money'.

It is my view that incoherence is usually the result of the same mechanism as derailment, and represents severe derailment. This is consistent with the view of others that mild forms of incoherence are rare (not to mention, impossible by definition).

Some authors (Kaplan and Saddock, 1991) give definitions of both incoherence and word salad. These are the same phenomena and it is recommended that only one be used.

Incoherence can sound like dysphasia and thorough neurological investigation is mandatory in the event of sudden onset. Intoxication with a wide range of agents needs to be excluded.

Incoherence due to psychiatric disorders is not common. It is evidence of severe disorder. One might expect incoherence to be most commonly encountered in schizophrenia. Almost certainly that would have been the case in the past. The symptoms observed in schizophrenia in recent times seem to be less severe than they were in the past – there is speculation that the disease is changing – there is no doubt that the care of schizophrenic people is better and more immediate than formerly. It may

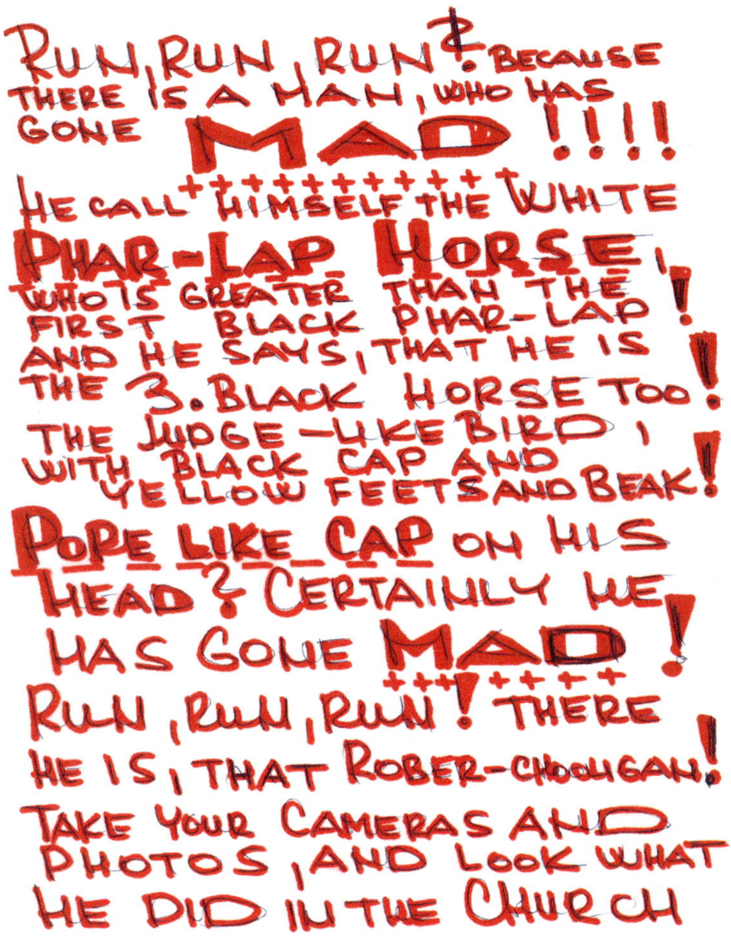

RUN, RUN, RUN? BECAUSE
THERE IS A MAN, WHO HAS
GONE MAD !!!!
HE CALL+ ++++++++ THE WHITE
PHAR-LAP HORSE,
WHO IS GREATER THAN THE
FIRST BLACK PHAR-LAP !
AND HE SAYS, THAT HE IS
THE 3. BLACK HORSE TOO!
THE JUDGE-LIKE BIRD,
WITH BLACK CAP AND
YELLOW FEETS AND BEAK!
POPE LIKE CAP ON HIS
HEAD? CERTAINLY HE
HAS GONE MAD !
RUN, RUN, RUN! +++ ++++ THERE
HE IS, THAT ROBER-CHOOLIGAN!
TAKE YOUR CAMERAS AND
PHOTOS, AND LOOK WHAT
HE DID IN THE CHURCH

Figure 22. This piece of writing was left anonymously at a politician's office. No details are known of the writer.

It is an example of incoherent thought disorder. There are two references to 'mad', which may suggest a measure of insight, and there is mention of 'cameras' which may suggest a paranoid delusion.

be that incoherence is just as often encountered in mania. This can be a rapidly escalating disorder and incoherence can certainly manifest. Presumably it could be possible with a patient at about the point of depressive stupor, but incoherence has not been observed by the author in depression.

Neologism

New words are invented by the speaker, words are distorted, or standard words are used in an idiosyncratic manner (Rifkin, 1991).

Andreasen (1979) reserved the term neologism for those items, the derivation of which cannot be understood, e.g., 'a tavro' and 'replaper'. She suggested a separate category of 'word approximations' for new words developed by the conventional rules of word formation, e.g., 'handshoes' (gloves). Under this heading she also included the idiosyncratic use of words, such as when a patient used the word 'vessel' in an unusual manner – for him, a watch was a 'time vessel', the stomach was a 'food vessel' and the television was a 'news vessel'.

Distortion of certain words may occur. A patient with schizophrenia mispronounced the name of the city, Melbourne. She said (phonetically), 'Melvern'. This was the only word she mispronounced. She could pronounce the word Melbourne correctly, she acknowledged that she pronounced it differently to others, but she could not give a reason for so doing.

At this time, in clinical practice there is no clear benefit from distinguishing between new words, word approximations and word distortions (research may change this position), and it is recommended that they be grouped together as forms of neologism.

A remarkable feature is that the patient seems unaware that neologisms lack meaning to the listener. When the examiner stops the conversation and asks what a particular neologism means, the patient usually still shows no surprise, but depending on the degree of thought disorder, may answer as if defining a standard word.

It is possible that neologisms could occur as a feature of an organic condition. If a patient presented with frequent neologisms the thought would be incoherent and dysphasias would need to be excluded. This is rarely the case, neologisms usually present as single, stark, curious specimens in an otherwise less remarkable stream, and accordingly, it is rarely difficult to distinguish them from dysphasia. Neologisms are relatively rare, occurring in a very small percentage of those people suffering schizophrenia or mania. In mania they are a function of the increased speed of thought and can be expected to disappear with resolution of the episode. In schizophrenia, the impression is they are a sign of severe illness and may indicate a less favourable prognosis.

Blocking (thought block)

Interruption in the train of speech/thought before the thought is completed. Patients stop speaking, then after a period of seconds to minutes, indicate that they are unable to remember what they had intended to say.

Blocking may give rise to the delusion that thoughts have been withdrawn from the head (thought withdrawal).

Blocking is over-diagnosed. It is a rare phenomenon. It is included here in part to emphasise the point that it should only be identified if it occurs in mid-thought and if the patient volunteers or admits on questioning that the thought was lost.

In rare instances thought blocking may be experienced as a single, or series of threatening events, in which case the presence of this symptom may be clearly declared or complained of by the patient.

True thought blocking must be distinguished from the benign form that occurs in normal individuals. In this form the symptom arises as an isolated event, more often when we are tired or distracted by other thoughts. Care must also be taken not to make the diagnosis when patients are simply distracted by delusions or hallucinations.

It is seen in schizophrenia. In mania there may be loss of a train of thought, but the patient does not appear concerned that the topic has been lost – rather, they pass on to the topic which distracted their thinking.

Perseveration and echolalia

Perseveration is the repetitive expression of a particular word, phrase or concept during the course of speech.

The example of perseveration given by both Andreasen (1979) and Rifkin (1991) is, 'I think I'll put on my hat, my hat, my hat, my hat.' Perseveration of concept/topic is often less obvious (see Figure 23).

Echolalia is the pathological repeating of the words or phrases of one person by another. It is often with a mocking or staccato intonation. Such delivery can be misinterpreted as being designed to give offence. Other evidence indicates there is no such intention.

Perseveration and echolalia are presented together because the central feature of both is repetition (one of one's own words, and the other of another's). Future research may reveal different processes, in which case they should again be considered separately.

Perseveration occurs in organic conditions and such conditions must be excluded. When both forms are considered (word and concept/topic) it occurs not infrequently in both schizophrenia and mania.

Echolalia occurs in organic conditions, particularly in dementia complicated by dysphasia and in some individuals with mental retardation. It can occur in schizophrenia and mania (more frequently in severe cases).

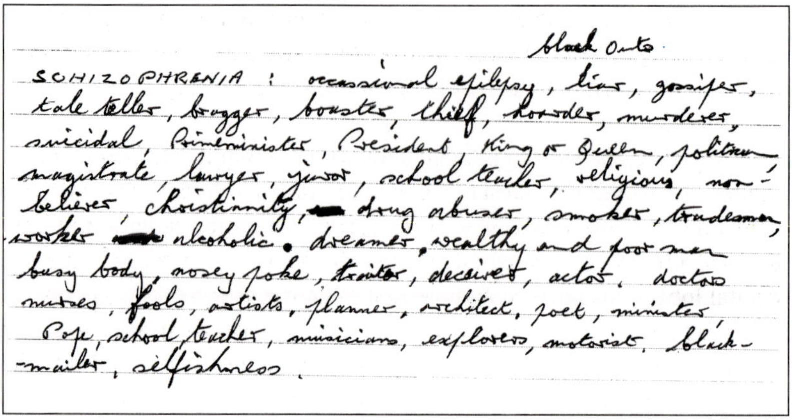

Figure 23. This example was written by a twenty-two-year old university student who had been diagnosed as suffering from schizophrenia. He rejected the suggestion that he was mentally ill. He studied a standard English dictionary and compiled the above list. At a subsequent meeting with his doctor he presented this document as 'proof' that he did not have schizophrenia. Poignantly, on the contrary, his 'proof' served to further substantiate the diagnosis.

This composition is replete with derailment and perseveration. It is not clear why the derailment occurred from 'SCHIZOPHRENIA' onto the topic of epilepsy, and then onto the word 'liar'. Once on the topic of speakers he perseverated, generating the list – 'gossiper, tale teller, bragger, boaster'.

At another point he lists heads of state and government positions – 'Primeminister, President, King or Queen, politician', before derailing through a number of steps to the word 'christianity'.

The original was written in blue ink. At the end, after a list of more than a dozen vocations the patient added, in black ink (apparently some time later), the noun 'selfishness' – which is not a vocation.

Taken as an argument against the diagnosis of schizophrenia, this composition is an example of poverty of content of thought or incoherence. There are many words but due to derailment and perseveration the counter argument is not structured, cohesive or persuasive.

Poverty of thought (speech)

Speech is decreased in amount, is not spontaneous and consists mainly of brief and unelaborated responses to questions.

Replies may be monosyllabic, and some questions may be left unanswered altogether. The interviewer will have to keep prompting and asking for elaboration. The interview can be frustrating.

For example, consider the response to the question, 'Do you have children?'. If the answer is in the affirmative, the person without psychopathology usually responds immediately, stating the affirmative case and usually giving the number and sex, often the ages and sometimes the names, of the children. Where there is poverty of thought the patient may not make any response when the question is first asked. The interviewer may feel the need to ask the question a second time and after a long pause the patient may answer, '...Yes...', often without any supplementary information as to number, ages or names. Even the word yes may be mumbled or otherwise unclear.

In the presence of apparent poverty of thought, the two main organic conditions that deserve consideration are hypothyroidism and dementia/frontal lobe damage. Slowness of mentation (and other physiological processes) is well established in hypothyroidism; in dementia/frontal lobe damage there may be lack of conversation due to apathy.

Depression must be considered. A core feature of depression may be slowness in the production of thoughts (psychomotor retardation). This reverts to normal with resolution of the episode.

Poverty of thought is common in chronic schizophrenia, where it is often accompanied by other 'negative' symptoms. Here it appears to be due to abnormality in mesocortical projections and/or prefrontal cortical cellular architecture and is unlikely to spontaneously revert.

Poverty of content

The subject talks freely, fluently and coherently, but in spite of an adequate number of words, little information is given, due to vagueness, stereotyped phrases or thought disorder such as derailment (Figures 23, 24, **25**).

Wing *et al.* (1974) advise poverty of content must be differentiated from incoherence and flight (but these are the only types of formal thought disorder they recognise). Andreasen (1979) advises to differentiate from circumstantiality, where the patient gives a wealth of detail.

Poverty of content is often the result of derailment. Often this is subtle and the interviewer is expecting the patient to get to the point and convey some significant information at any moment. But that moment does not come. If poverty of content is the result of derailment, the record of interview should mention both – these are not mutually exclusive terms.

When the patient is talking of yoga, spiritualism or quasi-philosophical matters, poverty of content of thought is frequently present. The patient is attracted to these topics partly because the call for critical, logical thought is less pressing in such discussions. They may find comfort in belonging to such interest groups. At interview, when the patient is talking about these topics, derailment (for example) is more difficult to identify.

The test of whether there is poverty of content is to listen to the patient talk on a topic for a brief period and then attempt to make a summary. The product of normal thought processes can be reduced to a

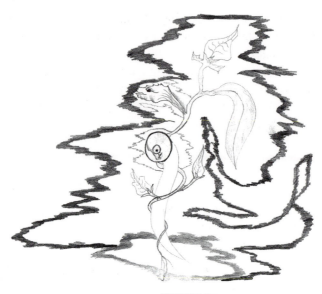

"AN ABSTRACT LIVING VIEW"

Figure 24. This drawing was made by a young psychotic man. His parents brought him to hospital because they could not understand what he was saying, he had unexpectedly stopped going to work and was spending most of the day alone in his room.

On examination there was poverty of content of thought. He could not give a clear explanation of his parents' concerns or why he had stopped going to work. He spoke about the meaning of life and said that 'society' was going to be 'reorganised'.

A few days after admission the patient presented this drawing to staff. He indicated that it was the answer to all questions, including those about the recent events of his life and the future of the human race. Initially, he could not describe or give a name to his drawing. The following day he called it 'An Abstract Living View'.

The drawing depicts a plant with roots, stems and leaves, possibly extending from a seed. There is the head of what may be a supernatural being arising from a point on a stem.

Apparently similar creations are produced by visual artists (particularly the surrealists) who break the rules, juxtapose unexpectedly and express ideas symbolically.

To the person untrained in art criticism (and perhaps also to those who are trained in art criticism) the difference between the work of the visual artist and the thought disordered person is not so much in the work but in the explanation of the meaning of the work. The visual artist may purposefully depart from realism while the thought disordered person departs from realism unintentionally.

Visual artists will be able to give a cogent explanation of the meaning of their work; the thought disordered person will usually give, at best, a vague explanation.

A difference becomes clearer in the long term. The visual artist continues to produce and there is stylistic progression over time. The thought disordered person who produces an interesting piece, usually does not continue to generate work. This is because thought disorder makes organization of resources difficult and because this symptom is usually accompanied by others (disorders of affect and volition) which militate against productivity. In those cases in which a thought disordered person continues to produce, there is little stylistic progression, rather, there is indefinite repetition (perseveration [see Shallice, 1988]) in subject and style.

pithy summary. Where there is poverty of content, it is not that many words can be reduced to a short summary, but that there is almost no information to summarise.

Poverty of content may be difficult to differentiate from the output of the particularly verbose normal individual or the narcissistic individual. It may occur with intoxication of various types. It is most common in schizophrenia but may occur in mania.

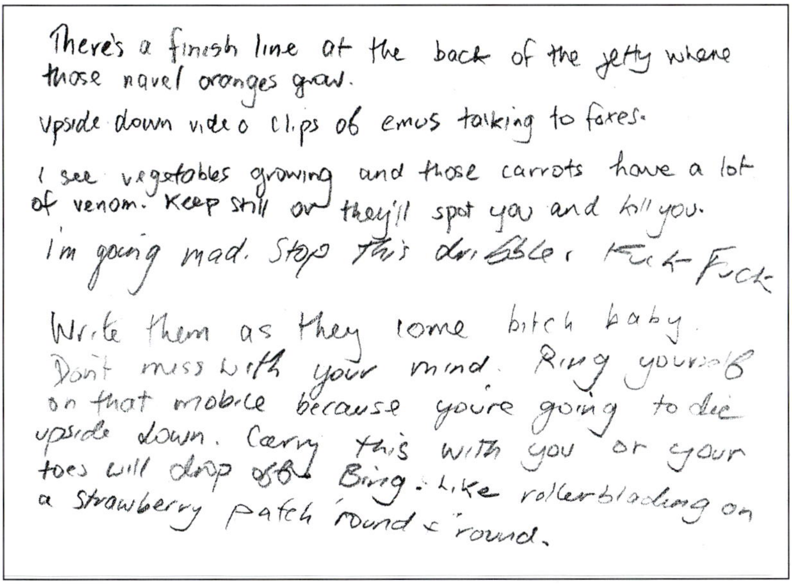
There's a finish line at the back of the jetty where
those navel oranges grow.
Upside down video clips of emus talking to foxes.
I see vegetables growing and those carrots have a lot
of venom. Keep still or they'll spot you and kill you.
I'm going mad. Stop this dribble. Fuck Fuck

Write them as they come bitch baby.
Don't miss with your mind. Ring yourself
on that mobile because you're going to die
upside down. Carry this with you or your
toes will drop off. Bring. Like rollerblading on
a strawberry patch round & round.

Figure 25. These lines were written by a young woman during a manic phase. They look like two verses of poetry – but that was coincidental, not intentional. Instead, these were thought 'grabs' as pressured thoughts raced through her mind. The reader gets a sense of the pressure – and that the patient has had to scrawl down this nonsense to relieve that pressure. This is flight of ideas – in the first one and a half lines the idea changed from 'finish line' to 'jetty' (perhaps fishing line and jetty) to 'navel oranges' (perhaps jetty and navy). It is difficult to see the connections between ideas in most instances.

This young person had insight ('I'm going mad') and found the experience distressing ('Fuck, Fuck') – so much for mania being a happy state.

There is pressure of thought and flight of ideas – but this example has been included as an example of poverty of content – arising out of mania. (Poverty of content is most commonly observed in schizophrenia.) This is close to incoherence, but in my opinion, that degree of disorder has not been demonstrated (although such judgments are matters of opinion, and others may disagree). There is evidence that thinking was taking place, standard words are used and proper sentences with objects, subjects and verbs are constructed – but no cohesive, sensible message is transmitted.

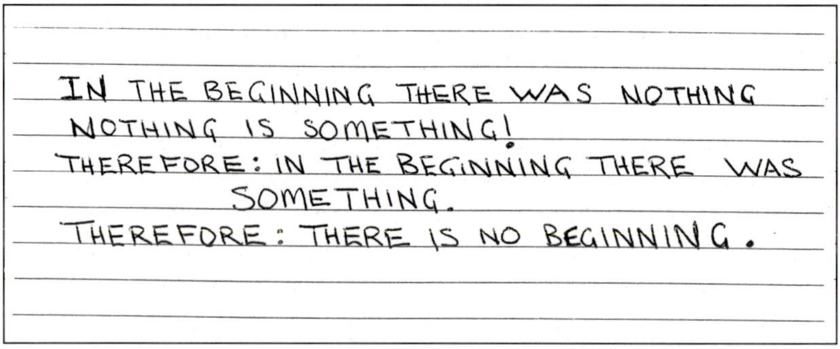

IN THE BEGINNING THERE WAS NOTHING
NOTHING IS SOMETHING!
THEREFORE: IN THE BEGINNING THERE WAS
        SOMETHING.
THEREFORE: THERE IS NO BEGINNING.

Figure 26. This passage was written by a young man during an acute episode of schizoaffective disorder. During this episode he carried a writing pad and made notes throughout the day. This appeared to be because he was overactive, but it may also have helped him control disorganised thinking.

The passage is an example of illogicality of thought. Challenging, iconoclastic statements are not uncommon in mood elevated states – but mood elevation was not the basis of this statement as it was verbally repeated by the patient during periods of euthymia.

Illogicality

Illogicality is present where there are erroneous conclusions or internal contradictions in thinking. Figure 26, 27.

This category is included for its contribution to the reader's knowledge base and confidence. Illogicality is a difficult category, which survives in disputed territory between disorders of thought form and content. The term illogicality is rarely essential for good clinical practice and often confuses rather than clarifies discussions.

For illogicality the patient must make a number of statements, and at least one must contradict another. Thus, the content of what the patient is saying/thinking must be considered. Most often the patient is psychotic

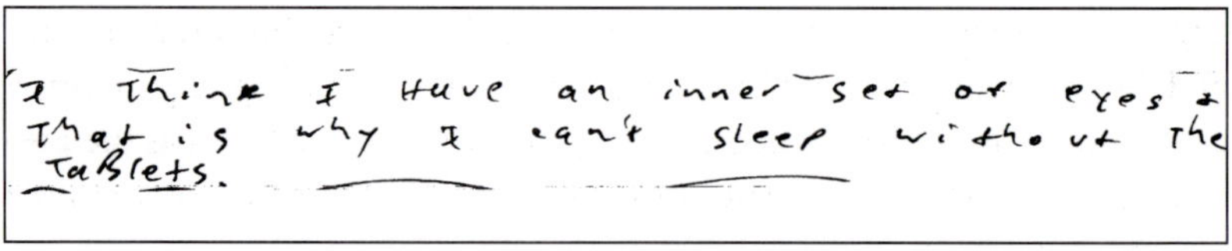

I think I have an inner set of eyes + That is why I can't sleep without the Tablets.

Figure 27. This was written by a young man who suffered schizophrenia. Here he states that he needs tablets to sleep because he has 'an inner set of eyes'. This may be interpreted as the statement of a delusion.

An alternative, speculative explanation for this statement involves formal thought disorder – the patient has found that he cannot sleep without medication – he knows that one's eyes close when one sleeps – and as he closes his eyes and attempts, but cannot sleep, he makes the illogical conclusion that he has a second pair of eyes which will not close.

and is reporting a delusion. It is easy to pick up on the disorder of content; what is often missed is that there is also illogicality which is a disorder of the form of thought.

A patient believed that there were aliens on earth. He stated that when they looked at normal human beings, the normal human beings immediately burst into flames and died. He further stated that he knew this because he was a normal human being and he had been looked at by aliens on at least a dozen occasions. The disorder of content is not difficult to spot. But we are interested here in the illogicality. The patient stated that he was a normal human being (there would not have been any illogicality if he had claimed to be a God with special powers). If his belief had been correct, he should have been burnt to death. He was not dead – he was alive and talking. The logical impossibility, when pointed out, did not concern him, nor was his belief modified to avoid the illogicality.

As delusions are beliefs held in spite of evidence to the contrary, it can be argued that where there is a delusion there is illogical thinking. But for current purposes the illogicality needs to be an intrinsic feature of the thought processes of the patient.

Intoxication needs to be excluded. The thoughts of normal people reveal a good deal of illogicality, when closely scrutinised. Nevertheless, when clear examples of illogicality occur they excite interest and suggest delusional disorder and schizophrenia.

Content

Disorders of content of thought have a profound effect on the mental life of the individual, influencing subsequent thinking, feeling and behaviour. They are usually immediately apparent at interview and often constitute the presenting complaint. When a patient presents with a complaint which is secondary to a disorder of content of thought, such as insomnia secondary to the belief that attack by an enemy is imminent, both the primary and the secondary problems may be listed under the heading of presenting complaint. Alternatively, the secondary problem may be listed as the presenting complaint while the primary problem is listed in the history of the presenting complaint.

Disorders of content of thought are usually mentioned under the heading of presenting complaint (or history thereof), but as there is also provision for mention of content of thought under the heading of mental state, interviewers are sometimes uncertain about emphasis and repetition. The following is an acceptable arrangement. Complete details are given under the heading of presenting complaint (or history thereof). These are followed by the rest of the history. In the mental state, under the heading of content of thought, some brief reminding details are offered and the reader or listener is referred back to the presenting complaint for the complete account.

When one individual believes one thing and a second believes the opposite, the scene is set for conflict. Individuals with disorders of the content of thought often believe things that the interviewer does not believe. For example, a patient may believe he is being watched by people from another country, political system or planet. The interviewer, wishing to avoid conflict, may be concerned about what to answer if asked whether he or she 'believes' what the patient is saying. In practice, it is surprising how infrequently a patient with a false belief actually confronts the interviewer with the question, 'Do you believe me?'. Often the patient is so occupied with the thoughts, that little interest is shown in what the interviewer believes. In other cases, the patient has argued the issue with numerous people before coming to the interview and no longer expects others to share his or her beliefs. However, when the question does arise, it is appropriate to indicate that the interviewer believes the patient, but not the belief, for example, 'I believe you believe what you are saying'. (This is the standard response, but can sound like glib trickery.) Once asked this question, the interviewer has the opportunity to strengthen the relationship, with, for example, 'I know you're telling me the truth as you see it, but I'm not sure I can agree, because...'. [The advantages of this response are: the statement by the interviewer that the patient is telling the truth, which is polite and positive; it gets away from the complicated issue of 'belief'; and it respectfully invites the patient to explore other explanations. The point of this invitation is not so much a therapeutic endeavour (it is unlikely that, in the early stages at least, a patient will be persuaded away from a delusional conviction), but a means of assessing the extent of the delusional system and the strength of the conviction.]

Delusion

Delusions are false beliefs that are sustained despite evidence to the contrary. They are out of keeping with the patient's social, cultural and educational background.

The following are useful terms that can be applied to delusions. Some apply to the subject matter of the delusion, such as parts of the patient's body (somatic), harassment (persecutory) or self-accusation (guilt). Others refer to other aspects of the mental state (mood-congruent and mood-incongruent) and yet others refer to the degree of organisation within the

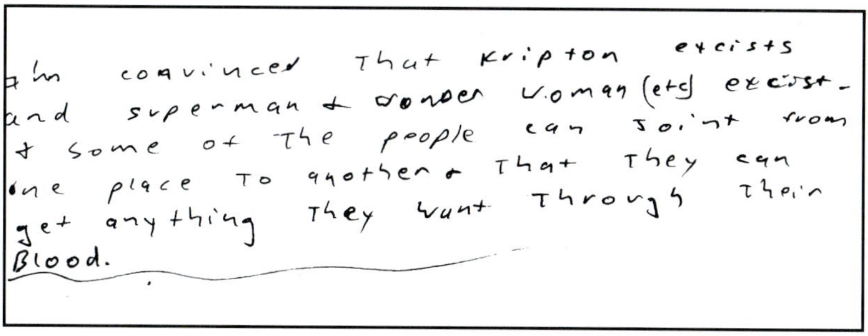

Figure 28. Here the previous patient is expressing a bizarre delusion (that the fictional characters Superman and Wonder Woman exist) – he then adds the further belief that these characters can 'get what they want' (presumably nutrition, perhaps other things) 'through their blood'. This further belief could be regarded as a second delusion, but it would be better to simply regard the first delusion as being somewhat elaborated. This passage lacks sufficient complexity and influence over the patient's life to qualify as a systematized delusion.

delusion (systematised). Except for mood-congruent and mood-incongruent, these are not mutually exclusive terms. No delusion is pathognomonic of any mental disorder – any can occur in any psychotic disorder – but some are more suggestive of certain disorders than others and will be mentioned as they arise. No ranking in importance is possible or intended.

Bizarre delusions

These delusions are absurd, implausible and factually not possible. The subject matter often includes the supernatural or space creatures (Figure 28). The term was not used in the older descriptions of psychopathology but became prominent with recent versions of the DSM. Bizarre delusions are found in schizophrenia, mood disorder and organic states.

Grandiose delusions

These are delusions of ability, beauty, influence or importance – they are beliefs that are inconsistent with the patient's assets (Figure 29, 30). They are frequently present in mood elevation, as occurs in mania, and intoxication with stimulants and euphoriants. They are also a feature of paranoid conditions.

Persecutory delusions

These are delusions of being harassed, persecuted, cheated, threatened, watched or bugged (Figure 29). These delusions may involve God and/or the devil, space creatures, spies, communists, religious groups to which

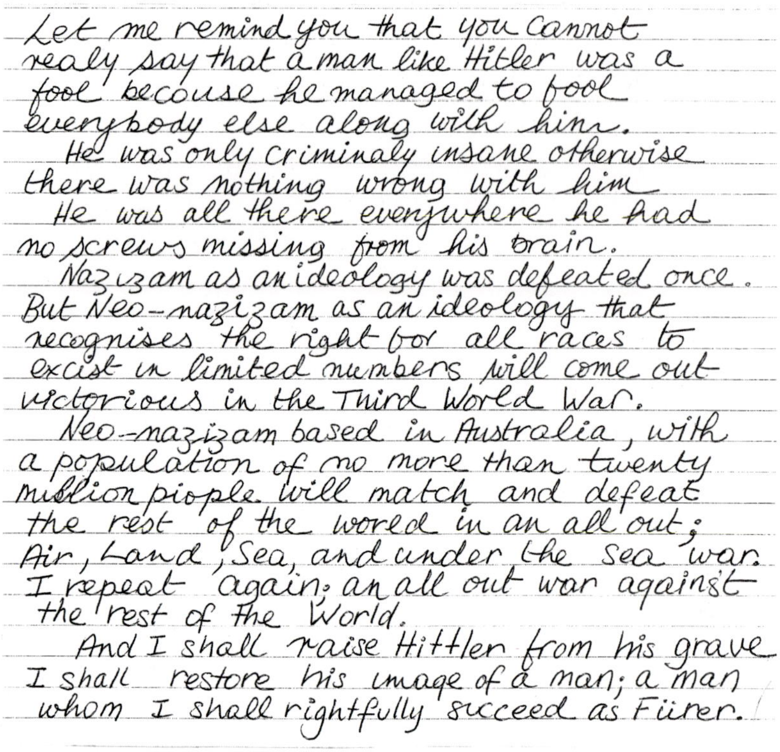

Let me remind you that you cannot
realy say that a man like Hitler was a
fool becouse he managed to fool
everybody else along with him.
    He was only criminaly insane otherwise
there was nothing wrong with him
    He was all there evenjwhere he had
no screws missing from his brain.
    Nazizam as an ideology was defeated once.
But Neo-nazizam as an ideology that
recognises the right for all races to
excist in limited numbers will come out
victorious in the Third World War.
    Neo-nazizam based in Australia, with
a population of no more than twenty
million piople will match and defeat
the rest of the worled in an all out;
Air, Land, Sea, and under the sea war.
I repeat again; an all out war against
the rest of the World.
    And I shall raise Hittler from his grave
I shall restore his image of a man; a man
whom I shall rightfully succeed as Fürer.

Figure 29. This document was written by a man whose first language was not English. In such circumstances, it is almost impossible to detect formal thought disorder with certainty.

The disorder of content of thought, however, is inescapable. The following is a grandiose delusion – 'AND I SHALL RAISE HITTLER FROM HIS GRAVE I SHALL RESTORE HIS IMAGE OF A MAN; A MAN WHOM I SHALL RIGHTFULLY SUCCEED AS FURER'.

the patient does not belong, homosexuals or neighbours. They are found in all forms of psychosis (Figure 30).

Delusions of reference

Things that other people do or have done are believed to refer to the patient (Figure 31). Items in print, the things said on radio or television or actions of people in the street (such as coughing, covering the mouth or crossing the road) are believed to have special meaning – usually telling the patient or other people of the patient's past or present deeds. The patient is frequently 'innocent' of these deeds or attributes. For example, the coughing of a stranger in a shop may be taken as a communication to others in the shop that the patient is a child molester or homosexual when neither is the case.

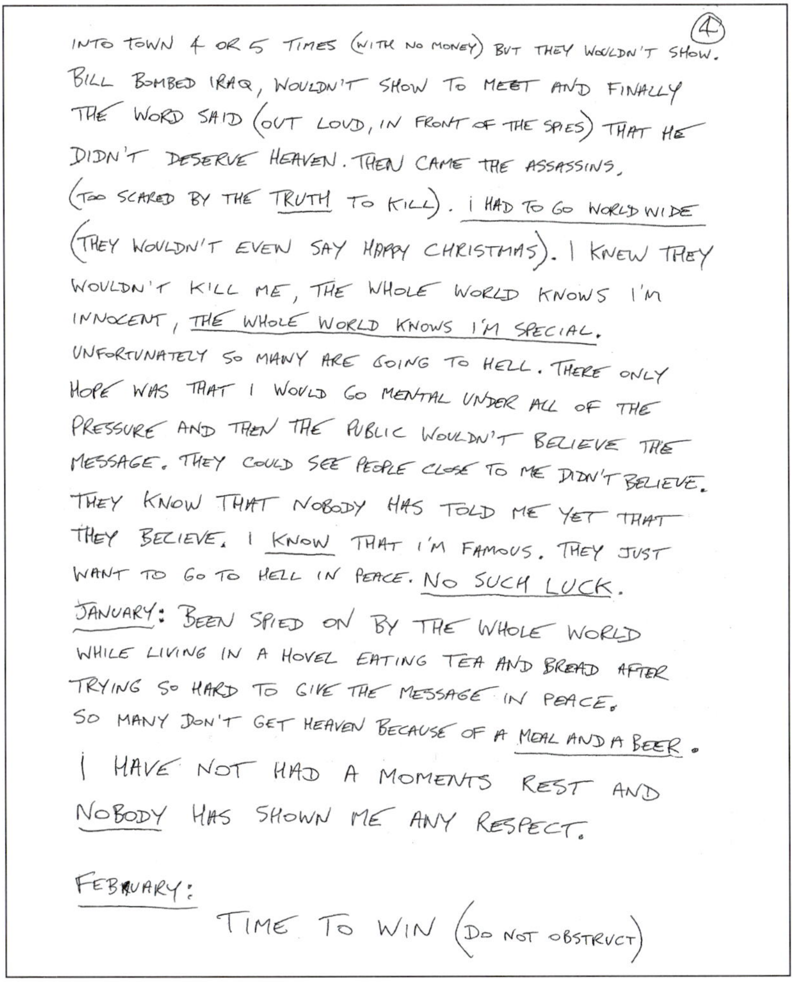

INTO TOWN 4 OR 5 TIMES (WITH NO MONEY) BUT THEY WOULDN'T SHOW. ④
BILL BOMBED IRAQ, WOULDN'T SHOW TO MEET AND FINALLY
THE WORD SAID (OUT LOUD, IN FRONT OF THE SPIES) THAT HE
DIDN'T DESERVE HEAVEN. THEN CAME THE ASSASSINS,
(TOO SCARED BY THE TRUTH TO KILL). i HAD TO GO WORLDWIDE
(THEY WOULDN'T EVEN SAY HAPPY CHRISTMAS). I KNEW THEY
WOULDN'T KILL ME, THE WHOLE WORLD KNOWS I'M
INNOCENT, THE WHOLE WORLD KNOWS I'M SPECIAL.
UNFORTUNATELY SO MANY ARE GOING TO HELL. THERE ONLY
HOPE WAS THAT I WOULD GO MENTAL UNDER ALL OF THE
PRESSURE AND THEN THE PUBLIC WOULDN'T BELIEVE THE
MESSAGE. THEY COULD SEE PEOPLE CLOSE TO ME DIDN'T BELIEVE.
THEY KNOW THAT NOBODY HAS TOLD ME YET THAT
THEY BELIEVE. I KNOW THAT I'M FAMOUS. THEY JUST
WANT TO GO TO HELL IN PEACE. NO SUCH LUCK.
JANUARY: BEEN SPIED ON BY THE WHOLE WORLD
WHILE LIVING IN A HOVEL EATING TEA AND BREAD AFTER
TRYING SO HARD TO GIVE THE MESSAGE IN PEACE.
SO MANY DON'T GET HEAVEN BECAUSE OF A MEAL AND A BEER.
I HAVE NOT HAD A MOMENTS REST AND
NOBODY HAS SHOWN ME ANY RESPECT.

FEBRUARY:
TIME TO WIN (DO NOT OBSTRUCT)

Figure 30. This was written by a middle-aged man who suffered from paranoid schizophrenia. He died by suicide in prison. After many years of trying to convince others of his mission to spread peace, he assaulted an acquaintance and was convicted.

This short passage has much psychopathology. The patient claims that he was being spied upon. This is a sign of persecutory delusion. The belief that one is being spied upon or bugged is a common persecutory theme.

There is also grandiosity. The patient believed that the whole world was aware of him and that he was famous. Paranoid conditions (by which is meant paranoid schizophrenia and delusional disorder of persecutory type) frequently manifest grandiose features. Such claims could also be a feature of mood elevation and extreme narcissistic personality disorder.

There is evidence of formal thought disorder. Immediately after the grandiose statement that he 'had to go world wide' the patient derails onto a statement that 'they wouldn't even say Happy Christmas'. The above is an extract, but even from the original document it was not clear to whom the patient was referring. The arguement does not flow logically, but is a series of strong, loosely connected assertions.

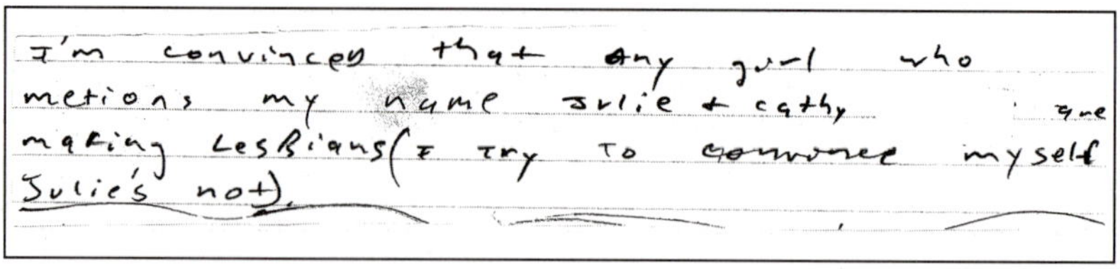

I'm convinced that any girl who metions my name Julie + Cathy are mating Lesbians (I try to convince myself Julie's not).

Figure 31. This piece of writing contains formal thought disorder. It would therefore be impossible to be certain of the intended message of this small sample without further information.

'Julie' and 'Cathy' were characters in a long-running television series.

The patient, who had a common first name, was infatuated with both of these characters, particularly 'Julie'. He believed that whenever a female said his first name, even when referring to another person of the same name, that they were indicating to him, information concerning the sexual preferences of 'Cathy' and 'Julie'.

This passage contains a delusion of reference, albeit complicated by derailment.

Delusions of reference are found in all forms of psychosis. In mania, they usually refer to the patient's superior qualities, and in schizophrenia they are often threatening.

Ideas of reference may occur in psychotic and non-psychotic disorders. They lack delusional strength. Patients can be convinced that although 'it seems like it', the actions of others do not, in fact, refer to them.

Ideas of reference may occur in social phobia, where the patient has the experience that others seem to be aware of his or her discomfort. However, the term is rarely used in non-psychotic conditions because of a strong association with psychotic conditions such as schizophrenia.

Delusions of control

Patients believe some external force is controlling their thoughts, feelings or movements, and they may complain of loss of autonomy or feeling like a robot. They may state that they do not 'will' certain of their thoughts or actions, it is as if these are 'willed' by an external force. This does not include being influenced by a person, idea or God, unless there is loss of control to this external force.

There are three named delusions which are often listed separately but which can be conveniently placed under the heading of delusions of control. These all have the patients thinking processes as their focus.

Thought withdrawal

The delusion that thoughts are being removed from the head. This is usually secondary to the disorder of the form of thought called thought blocking.

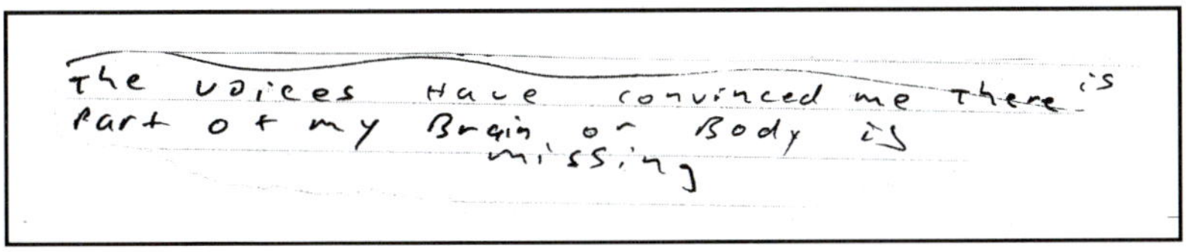

The voices Have convinced me there's part of my Brain or Body is missing]

Figure 32. The impression is not that 'the voices' told the patient that part of his brain or body was missing. It would be unwise to draw firm conclusions from such a tiny fragment of writing, but a number of explanations could be explored. It may be that the patient was aware that his hallucinations were symptoms of illness and he therefore concluded that this was the result of a missing physical structure. In similar circumstances, some authorities would use the term 'loosening of the boundaries of the self' and Bleuler's description of 'splitting of personality fragments' (p. 298) may be relevant. Whatever the explanation, this sentence is best conceptualized as a nihilistic delusion.

There is no doubt, the belief that part of one's brain or body is missing would be bewildering and frightening.

Thought insertion

The delusion that thoughts are being inserted into the mind by external forces. In thought blocking (which leads to the delusion of thought withdrawal) there is an actual experience by the patient of their thoughts stopping – the sudden cessation in speech and on occasions, a quizzical look on the face of the patient, can be observed. The nature of the experience leading to the delusion of thought insertion is less clear. In rare cases the patient will claim a sudden thought is not their own, but there is not a distinct term complimentary to thought blocking for this experience. Instead, in clinical practice, the term thought insertion is often applied to both the experience and the explanation (delusion).

Thought broadcasting

The delusion that the patient's thoughts can be heard by other people. A cautionary note – the belief is that the thoughts are actually heard by others – it is not simply that others know what the patient is thinking.

These three delusions could, with equal justification, have been collected under the heading of persecutory delusion. They occur in psychotic disorders.

Nihilistic delusion

The delusion that part of the self, the entire self, others or parts of the world do not exist or are in the process of ending (Figure 32). Nihilistic delusions are not common. When they do occur, one of the more common is that the patient is dead – that is, the patient believes himself or herself to be dead. Another is of poverty – severely depressed patients may believe they own no clothes or other possessions.

Characteristically, nihilistic delusions occur where there is depression of mood, such as in major depressive episode or in the depressed phase of schizoaffective disorder.

Somatic delusion

A delusion about a part of the patient's body, which may be bizarre, such as 'My brain has been replaced with a cat's liver', or non-bizarre such as the delusion that the patient has cancer of the rectum in spite of total absence of evidence. Some patients with somatic delusions are concerned that they emit a foul smell from their skin or orifices. Others believe their bodies (particularly their faces) are misshapen or ugly despite evidence to the contrary.

The belief of the person with anorexia nervosa that they are overweight may be held with delusional intensity, but this is accepted as an integral part of that condition and the term somatic delusion is not usually applied.

Hypochondriasis, according to current descriptions, is an overvalued belief that one is suffering a disease, but this belief is not held with delusional intensity. Somatic delusions are most usually encountered in schizophrenia, depression and delusional disorder.

In body dysmorphic disorder there is preoccupation with an imagined defect in appearance. This may lead to impairment of social functioning and the persuit of cosmetic surgery. If the thought is held with delusional intensity, however, the condition is classified as delusional disorder, somatic type.

Delusions of guilt

This term is applied when patients incorrectly believe they are guilty of, or responsible for, a certain act or set of actions which had a detrimental effect on others.

Many patients believe they have let their family or work mates down by being sick and unable to fulfil their role. This usually does not constitute a delusion of guilt. It is usually not held with delusional intensity – the patient will usually agree they are not responsible for their episodes of illness. Further, it is a fact that family and work mates will be inconvenienced by the patient's absence, thus there is usually no break with reality.

True delusions of guilt are not difficult to identify. One example is of a man who was severely depressed and suffering who attributed his current state to the fact that he had stolen some stamps for his stamp collection as a boy. He had psychomotor retardation and could not give a lucid account – it was not clear whether he believed that the stealing of the stamps set in train events which resulted in his present situation, or whether this was his punishment, handed down by some moral authority. He was suffering a delusion of guilt whatever his explanation and irrespective of whether he could give one.

Another example is a woman who believed she was responsible for a food crisis in Africa because she had been eating at expensive restaurants. She described a cascade of events beginning with her wastefulness, involving a recession in Australia and ending in a reduction in Australian financial support for developing economies.

Delusions of guilt occur most frequently in depressive disorder.

Delusional jealousy

Delusion that one's spouse or lover is unfaithful. This delusion often results in checking the partner's clothing for stains and other evidence, and may even result in the patient assaulting the partner.

Delusions of jealousy may be a feature of any psychosis. As the primary feature of what was called morbid or pathological jealousy (DSM-IV terminology is delusional disorder, jealous type) it is often related to chronic alcohol use.

Erotomanic delusions

Delusion that another person (usually a high-status person) is in love with the patient. This usually results in efforts to contact that person and this involves telephone calls, letters, gifts and personal contact. It may result in stalking and other forms of harassment. The advances are eventually rejected and legal consequences such as restraining orders and charges of assault may result. Knowing this condition exists, one sometimes notes accounts in the press which appear to have gone undiagnosed.

This condition is most frequently a feature of delusional disorder, erotomanic type.

Mood-congruent delusion

The term is only applied in mood disorder, where the delusion has mood-appropriate content. For example, a depressed person believes his family has been murdered, and cannot be reassured, even when they visit.

THE CASE FOR MARTIN BRYANT
16 October 1996

The reason Martin Bryant did what he did was because of an electronic mind control centre located under the 10th fairway at West Ryde Golf Links and I will proceed to prove it.

In 1985 when I was living in Queensland I started, all of a sudden, getting strange dreams of other people's experiences, usually sex, sometimes even before I was asleep. In one of these experiences I noticed lines through the image, like looking close to a television set, and being experienced in electronics, I realised it was being done electronically. This scared me so much that I left Queensland and went back to my parents place at xxxx Avenue, xxxxx. At that time I thought I was chosen because I used to hang around the stables at the Queensland Racecourses.

It took some eighteen months to figure out where it was coming from, and during this time, as my hatred grew, the dreams turned from sex dreams to dreams of carnage. Everything from being shot, stabbed, high speed traffic scares, to a bullet lodged in the brain for two days, so bad that I had to have a tooth pulled out.

Things were happening every day in the newspapers which terrified me, such as Tes De Brinkett being murdered, as I went to primary school with a girl named Brinkett who lived near the golf course in xxxx Crescent.

Eventually, I remembered, as a child playing in a drain pipe which ran under the 10th fairway and seeing a trap door open which frightened me and I ran away. This turns out to be an hallucination, and believe me, a nine-year-old shouldn't hallucinate.

I recalled the Wanda Beach Murders, and if you follow the creek past the house where these girls lived, it leads on to the golf links and eventually into a dam on the eleventh hole, next to the 10th fairway.

I went back to the 10th fairway to the drain pipe to see if this trap door was there, and now there is a grate about a meter across like a manhole in the middle of the 10th fairway (on a golf course mind you). I proceeded down the manhole into the drain pipe and noticed there were air vents, other smaller pipes, running from each side of the drain pipe about three quarters of the way up. I didn't find any trap door.

Somewhere around the time, Sydney changed over to natural gas (gas turbines most probably drive this machinery) which doesn't burn as violently, and they could no longer transmit high power things such as heart attacks, and bullets lodged in the brain.

When I got my next dole cheque I bought a sledge hammer and a few other tools. It was a Tuesday, Ladies Day, in October so I went onto the golf links and smashed a reticulation pipe which is for the sprinklers, as I thought this machine may be water cooled. That afternoon was the first I heard of the Stock Market Crash. After a few days they replaced the pipe so I started going back out there at night, smashing another five watering pipes, and chiseling at the dam wall as the entrance to this place may in fact be under the water. One night a policeman was waiting for me and he told me to lay down on the ground and put his gun in my back. He called on his radio for a police car, and I told him about the air vents in the drain pipe, and when the police car came he uncocked his gun while still holding it in my back. He had red hair and they took me to Ryde Police Station and after a short appearance in Court they took me to Long Bay Remand Centre. On the third Court appearance after about three weeks, I managed to escape custody. By now your right I was going insane, but I didn't care whether I lived or died.

I managed to get back on the dole and drifted around for a year or so, then went back out to the Golf Links to have another look for this trap door up the other direction from the grate. But when I got down the manhole, down past the air vents the drain pipe had been dammed up to about half way, probably with concrete so I couldn't get down to the air vents, although one air vent is right near the grate. It seems like the red haired policeman had been busy in his spare time.

One night I went back to the Golf Links and dug up 15 of the 18 greens (the other three were lit up near the club house) and it took them a couple of years to arrange the Greenough Axe Murders near Geraldton in WA. Now with Martin Bryant's case I was in Emerald Queensland when it happened. I was working, cotton chipping, with a bloke called Arthur and another There are examples of derailment: 'Everything from being shot, stabbed, high speed traffic scares, to a bullet lodged in the brain for two days, so bad that I had to have a tooth pulled out'. There is a delusion of reference: 'There is even a horse running around now called West Ryde King. Don't patronise me fellas'. It is interesting that this man 'dug up 15 of 18 golf course greens (the other three were litup near the club house)   ' Thus, although psychotic he was aware that what he was doing was illegal and he behaved rationally to escape detection.

called John, who looks exactly like the published photo of Martin Bryant (yes I can produce them).

I've been arrested since escaping, even spending three weeks at Newcastle lock up and Maitland Jail, but no record of my crimes concerning the golf links comes up, even though it made front page news of the Daily Mirror Country Edition, but only about page seven of the Sydney Edition. There is even a horse running around now called West Ryde King. Don't patronise me fellas. These murders are still occurring all over the world, the Rwanda Massacre, the trouble on the West Bank (this machine is located on the West Bank Dam, and the golf course is located between West Ryde and Meadowbank). They even blew up their own space shuttle Challenger.

While you're taking another month arguing whether to go and look at this drain pipe, Martin Bryant should be let out on bail. Governments aren't going to admit being involved in this. It's going to be a civilian mob to hold off the police while a couple of Powder Monkeys blow their way in.

This machine can transmit any disease a person has to any other person. Because of the sugar in your body, the nervous system is vibrated on to a frequency something like a quartz crystal in a digital watch which the two GB transmitter carried around the world back to itself to transmit and receive to you. Things like breast cancer, any cancer in fact, Alzheimer's disease, multiple sclerosis and they can transmit bad decisions to your doctor or bribe him with sex dreams, but they can't get me.

Figure 33. This document was written and widely distributed by an adult who is unknown to me. Martin Bryant murdered 35 people in one day in Tasmania.

Although there is formal thought disorder throughout this document, the message can be understood. It contains the bizarre delusion that there is 'an electric mind control center located under the 10th fairway at West Ryde Golf Links' and that it is being used to cause civil wars, aircraft accidents and disease. There is a well developed delusional system.

Mood-incongruent delusion

Again the term is only applied in mood disorder, where the content of the delusion has no association with mood. For example, a depressed person had a non-threatening delusion that his car had been used in the making of a film, although the film was made in USA, using American cars and the patient's car was of a type exclusively manufactured and sold in Australia.

Systematised delusions

Delusions united by a single theme – also referred to as a delusional system (Figure 33). Systematised delusions may be a feature of any psychosis – commonly found in delusional disorder and schizophrenia.

Obsession and compulsion

Obsessions are persistent, intrusive thoughts. They are usually distressing (such as the thought of killing a loved child) and recognised by the patient as a product of his or her mind and not imposed from outside. The patient attempts to suppress or neutralise these thoughts with other thoughts or actions.

Compulsions are repetitive, intentional behaviours that are performed in response to obsessions. As behaviours, their mention here under content of thought may be questioned. However, there are content of thought issues, with subjective pressure to perform the action, a desire to resist and the knowledge that the behaviour is excessive.

The above textbook description over-simplifies obsessions and compulsions. In clinical practice, the picture is usually complicated. While the connection between the fear of dirt/disease and frequent washing of the hands makes sense, the connection between many obsessions and compulsion is difficult to understand. In other cases a compulsion may exit without an accompanying obsession – an example was a man who had to turn the light on an off three times (irrespective of the time of day or night) when entering a room – he appeared to have no obsession whatsoever. While the purpose of a compulsion is to reduce the anxiety raised by the obsession, it too may cause distress (there may be a rationale for the compulsion, but it remains a silly, repetitive action with which the patient is uncomfortable). Thus, both resisting and submitting to both obsessions and compulsions may raise anxiety. And finally, the condition (in the case of obsessive–compulsive disorder) changes over time. After years of suffering, the patient may submit to the obsessions and compulsions. It becomes easier to give in to them than to resist them – that is, resisting these phenomena is anxiety provoking in the early stages, but when the condition is more entrenched and the patient is disabled, with submission the phenomena are less distressing.

True obsessions and compulsions, unaccompanied by other symptoms, are found only in obsessive–compulsive disorder. Obsession and compulsion-like symptoms may accompany other disorders such as schizophrenia and depressive disorder. These remit when the primary disorder abates.

Phobias

A phobia is a persistent, exaggerated and irrational fear of some specific stimulus, which results in a strong desire to avoid that stimulus. Exposure to the stimulus, *in vivo* or imagination, may result in a panic attack.

Agoraphobia

Agoraphobia, in literal terms, means fear of open market spaces. There are many clinical variations. Some authorities conceptualise agoraphobia as the fear of leaving safety – particularly the home. This may lead to the housebound housewife syndrome. For others the important issue may be the fear of being trapped in a place from which escape may be difficult or to which it may be difficult to bring help – this may lead to the avoidance of cramped queues at supermarkets or the chairs in hairdressing salons. There are two forms of agoraphobia – one is associated with panic disorder and the other is not.

In most cases there is avoidance of going out or into feared situations and supportive activity by family or friends.

When recording the disorder, in addition to the provocative issues, it is important to detail the presence or absence of panic, the degree of avoidance and the support provided by friends and relatives.

Social phobia

The essential feature is a persistent fear of one or more social situations in which the person could be scrutinised by others. The patient is concerned that he or she may behave in some way that will cause humiliation. The concerns and situations may be specific, such as being unable to continue while public speaking or choking on food while eating, or they may be more general concerns involving most social situations, such as saying something foolish or being unable to continue a conversation.

There may be avoidance of situations such as public speaking and eating in public.

Simple phobia

The essential feature is the persistent fear of a particular stimulus, other than fear of a panic attack (which is included in panic disorder) and fear of certain social situations (which are included in social phobia). Common examples include fear of insects, snakes, height and air travel.

As with other forms of anxiety, phobias may be associated with depressive features. In this case the questions to be considered include whether both anxiety disorder and depressive disorder are present (and if so, which preceded the other) or whether only one of these disorders is present, complicated by some features of the other.

Hypochondria

Hypochondria is an exaggerated concern regarding one's state of health. It is based not on actual organic pathology, but on inaccurate interpretation of normal physiological events or sensations, which are taken as evidence of physical illness. For example, breathlessness after walking up stairs may be taken as indicating heart disease, transient headache may be taken as indicating brain tumour. By convention, this is not a delusional phenomenon as the patient can be reassured, however, the fear/belief is notoriously persistent as is the consulting of doctors. The distinction from delusion is not always clear and the consulting of doctors approaches acting on a delusion.

Organic disease must be excluded. In hypochondriasis there are long-standing hypochondrical concerns. In some psychotic disorders, anxiety disorders and somatization disorders there may also be hypochondrical concerns which are not long-standing and are a feature of an acute episode. In delusional disorder of somatic type the patient cannot be convinced, even temporarily, that a physical abnormality does not exist.

Suicidal thoughts

Thoughts of suicide range from fleeting ideas in response to stressful events (which may occur in individuals without other psychopathology) through to determined, planned and finally executed acts (which are often, but not always, a feature of mental disorder). Social factors and suicidal behaviour by influential people in the life of the individual may also be important.

The interviewer makes an assessment of the risk of suicide in patients who present claiming suicidal thoughts and those patients who, by the nature of an existing mental disorder, are potentially at risk.

The interviewer should ask about suicidal thoughts, and make clear notes. Such notes are as much for the protection of the interviewer as for the patient. The best defence against the charge of negligence is to be able to prove that the time was taken to ask the appropriate questions and consider possibilities.

Generally speaking, at present, Western culture allows direct questions to be asked about suicidal thoughts without giving offence. Nevertheless, with some individuals, more progress may be made if the issue is approached gently. Examples include – 'You've got some problems at the moment. Have you ever wanted to escape from them? ... How would you do that? ... Have you ever thought of injuring yourself in any way?'; 'Do you ever feel that you deserve punishment? ... How would you do that?'; 'Have you ever thought of ending it all? ... What plans have you made?'; 'I don't mean to give offence in any way, but I am concerned about you. Some people, faced with these sorts of problems, think about suicide. Have you every thought of that sort of thing?'.

Talk (and the act) of suicide communicates distress. It does not necessarily imply a treatable psychiatric disorder. In individuals with Cluster B personality disorder (especially borderline, histrionic and antisocial type), it may be used as a way of threatening or demanding a particular response, such as admission to hospital, or some other requirement which is difficult to meet. It is known that some individuals with these personality types will die by suicide (some by accident during a suicidal gesture). Some apparently suicidal behaviour by overdose arises out of the desire for a period of rest or relief from problems. Suicide may be a feature of schizophrenia – in which case there may be evidence of recent distress and escalation of delusions, hallucinations and disorganised or bizarre behaviour. Suicide may be a feature of depressive disorder. In this case it may be preceded by subtle clues – the patient may not begin with thoughts of suicide, but spend time thinking about or missing deceased friends and relatives. Thoughts of guilt or the need for punishment demand action.

Homicidal thoughts

Medical defence experts now advise that in some jurisdictions doctors should make a record of having assessed not only suicidal but homicidal thinking in every examination. That is not my practice, but it may need to become so. Homicidal thinking is of two types.

Overt homicidal thinking

Here the patient talks openly of these thoughts

Non-psychotic overt homicidal thoughts

Non-psychotic here refers to the thinking process concerning the issue of homicide. A psychotic individual has many thoughts that are not disrupted by the psychosis – that is, psychosis rarely leads to problems with using the toilet, for example. Similarly, it is possible for a person with a psychotic illness to have non-psychotic thoughts about homicide.

Not infrequently, an individual presents to a health care professional stating that he or she has the inclination or intends to kill another person. This is usually in a setting of conflict and anger. It may be that the individual wants help with the anger, which can be a subjectively dysphoric experience.

Frequently, however, talk of homicide is presented to health care professionals for its manipulative value – to force the health system to provide admission or support, or to play an active part in resolution of a conflict. Depending on the resources and philosophy of the system, such activities may be beyond its role.

In the case of non-psychotic individuals talking of homicide, it is recommended that they be told that the law will hold them responsible for their actions. This can be delivered in a non-threatening manner – 'I can see that you are distressed, but you need to know that you do not have the sort of mental illness that will protect you, and the law will hold you responsible for anything you do'.

Those who are not psychotic and present to health care professionals with overt homicidal thoughts may be normal individuals under unusually severe stress. They are more usually drunk and may manifest a personality disorder. They may be patients whose ability to deal with stress has been reduced by a mental disorder (such people are still held responsible for their actions).

Psychotic overt homicidal thoughts

Psychotic here refers to the thinking process concerning the issue of homicide.

Rarely do psychotic individuals bring themselves to the health care professional with thoughts of homicide as a presenting complaint, but it does happen. More often the patient is brought in by others (police or family) who become aware of this thinking – or the individual presents with other problems and the homicidal thinking is discovered as a co-existing matter in the process of assessment.

Homicidal thoughts may be a feature of schizophrenia or delusional disorder. It will be necessary to take steps to protect the patient and the public.

Covert homicidal thinking

Here the patient does not talk openly about homicidal thoughts.

Non-psychotic covert homicidal thoughts

There is little place for mental health services. If this thinking is discovered the health professional should advise the patient that they will be held responsible for their actions (see above) and discuss the matter with medical defence authorities and/or police (depending on the regional legal system).

Psychotic covert homicidal thoughts

That this thinking is kept secret suggests a level of awareness that the action is against the law and the patient may well – despite the existence of psychosis – therefore, be answerable at law. But this is a complicated area beyond the scope of this book.

Where covert psychotic thinking about homicide exists or is suspected, the health professional should take action to secure the safety of the patient and the public.

Such problems can arise with individuals suffering paranoid illnesses. A huge problem exists with depressed individuals who kill family members in murder–suicide events. Such people may consider the world a terrible place and form the intention to exit via suicide. There may be various justifications for murdering family members, perhaps to spare them the terrors of the world, perhaps to conduct them to a better place, perhaps to take them as company. In such cases the diagnosis of depression may not be apparent and help may not be provided. The best that can be done is to remain alert to the possibility, treat depression energetically, and raise the alarm with family and perhaps police, where risk is considered present. (That is not to contend that all murder–suicide is the result of depressive disorder.)

6. Perception

Perception is the process of transferring physical stimulation into psychological information. That part of the mental state which is placed under the heading of 'perception' exemplifies the difficulties of classifying mental phenomena. The most often reported 'disorder of perception' is hallucination. By definition an hallucination is 'not associated with external stimuli', but by the earlier cited definition, perception involves the 'process of transferring physical stimulation'. It can be argued that hallucinations have nothing to do with perception, but there is insufficient present knowledge to justify alteration of the conventional system of classification.

A case can be made, however, for adding depersonalisation and delusional mood to the phenomena under the heading of perception.

Depersonalisation and derealization

Depersonalisation involves an alteration in the perception or experience of the self, in which the usual sense of one's own reality is temporarily lost or changed.

This can manifest as a feeling of detachment from and being an outside observer of one's mental processes or body, or of feeling like an automaton or as if in a dream. Patients may report that their movements or appearance in the mirror seem to be lifeless or subtly changed, but there is a lack of the delusional intensity found in delusions of control or somatic delusions.

Derealization is an alteration in the perception of one's surroundings so that the reality of the external world is lost – the world may appear two-dimensional as a stage set, sizes and shapes may be perceived as changed and others may appear mechanical or puppet like. The terms micropsia and macropsia have been applied when things appear smaller or larger than expected.

Suggested wording when seeking the phenomenon is offered by Wing *et al.* (1974) – 'Have you had the feeling that things around you are unreal?'.

Both derealization and depersonalisation are unpleasant experiences. Interestingly, they are said to be similar in many ways to certain intoxicated states, which are experienced as pleasurable. The difference may be one of autonomy – perhaps if the altered state is intentionally produced by the individual, he or she interprets it as pleasurable.

Depersonalisation and derealization may represent a 'normal' response to conditions of exhaustion and emotional shock. They may occur in a range of neurological, toxic and metabolic disorders. They may appear as an isolated psychiatric disorder under the designation depersonalisation disorder. They may appear as a feature of a wide range of psychiatric disorders including schizophrenia and mood, somatoform, anxiety and personality disorders.

Delusional mood

Delusional mood is present when a patient feels that familiar surroundings have changed in a puzzling way which may be difficult or impossible to describe, but which seems to be especially significant. The patient may simply say that everything seems odd and strange and that he or she cannot understand what is going on. This symptom may be experienced as ominous or threatening. The 'meaning' of these feelings may become clear to the subject when a delusion is formed.

Suggested wording when seeking the phenomenon is given by Wing *et al.* (1974) – 'Do you ever get the feeling that something odd is going on which you cannot explain?'.

This symptom is not described in detail in recent USA textbooks, although some describe 'perplexity', which is the same or a similar phenomenon. Clinical experience is that this is a useful and not uncommon observation in early schizophrenia. Clinically, this can be a difficult phenomenon to differentiate from depersonalisation/derealization. In delusional mood there is an inability on the part of the patient to 'explain' what is happening. This does not create a clear distinction as many people with depersonalisation also seek an explanation for their 'unreal' feelings.

Delusional mood, especially if suspicion is developing, suggests early schizophrenia. The term is generally not applied outside schizophrenia.

Heightened perception

Heightened perception is present when sounds seem unnaturally clear, loud or intense, colours appear more brilliant or beautiful, details of the environment seem to stand out in a particularly interesting way, or any sensation is experienced exceptionally vividly. Once the experience has passed, the subject may find it difficult to remember or describe.

This experience is reported in organic conditions, including drug use and temporal lobe epilepsy, and in the psychoses, schizophrenia and mania.

Changed perception

Changed perception includes changes in shape or size or change in the appearance of people.

Changed perceptions may be difficult to differentiate from derealization. Changed perceptions show more variation over time and may be interesting, pleasant or frightening. Derealization is usually continuously, moderately unpleasant, with some mild fluctuations.

Clinical experience suggests that changed perceptions may occur more commonly than is generally recognised. It is possible that when some psychotic individuals are difficult to engage in conversation, they are attending to continuously changing perception. As with heightened perception, patients find remembering or describing the phenomenon difficult, once it has ceased.

The diagnostic implications are as for heightened perceptions.

Hallucinations

Hallucinations are false sensory perceptions not associated with external stimuli. There may or may not be delusional interpretation of the hallucinatory experience. Hallucinations suggest psychosis only when there is impaired reality testing.

Hallucinations are generally experienced as being outside the patient – existing in the external world. The term pseudohallucination has been defined a number of ways; Wing *et al.* (1974) used the term for auditory hallucinations which are experienced as originating inside the head. Pseudohallucinations (by this definition) are often thought to have less pathological significance, but this has not been proven. Apart from this paragraph, in this text the term pseudohallucinations will not be used – that is, no distinction will be made between hallucinations inside and outside the head.

Examiners are sometimes reluctant to ask patients about the existence of hallucinations, concerned this may damage the patient–clinician relationship. There should be no such concerns and the clinician should proceed in a confident and professional manner. Just as the patient who presents to the GP with a lump in the base of the neck accepts a per rectum examination, so a patient presenting to a mental health clinician accepts examination of unexpected areas.

When the patient presents talking about hallucinations, there is no problem. A clinician may be concerned about a patient who has clear evidence of psychosis, such as disorder of the form and content of thought. If such a person is asked but does not have hallucinations the question will cause no problems and will soon be forgotten – but if the patient does have hallucinations he or she will be well served by the enquiry. Some may deny the experience and feign annoyance at the suggestion, but this lacks force and the suggestion does not damage the patient–clinician relationship. On the contrary, while the patient may continue to deny hallucinations for a time, he or she may be relieved to know the clinician is 'on the ball'.

In a case where there is no clear evidence of psychosis, the examiner may feel more comfortable if the question is softened – 'You've had some stressful experiences. When people experience a lot of stress they sometimes hear voices or other noises, or see things that they can't explain. Have you ever had anything like that, at all?'.

Investigators administering structured interviews and diagnostic instruments have expressed concern about the possibility of alienating people through questions about hallucinations. In these situations it is necessary to ask every question and the subjects may be members of the general public, generally without significant psychopathology. Accordingly, such interviewers are taught to say something like, 'Now, I would like to ask you some routine questions that we ask everyone. Do you ever seem to hear noises or voices when there is no one about?'

The following is a list of terms used to describe hallucinations. They are not mutually exclusive or arranged in any particular order.

Non-pathological hallucinations

Hallucinations may occur in circumstances where there is no significant psychopathology. Hypnogogic hallucinations occur when individuals are passing from the awake to the sleeping state. They usually take the form of the name being called and may cause the patient to leave bed to investigate. Hypnopompic hallucinations are less common, they occur as the individual is passing from the sleeping to the waking state. Hallucinations, often visual but also auditory, may accompany exhaustion and sleep deprivation, in which case they may be the result of dreaming extending into the waking state.

Bereaved people may have visual or auditory hallucinations of the deceased person. This is most common in the early stages of bereavement.

Persistence of, or distress from, such phenomena calls for comprehensive psychiatric examination.

Non-verbal auditory hallucinations

The patient hears noises other than words. Examples include clicking, buzzing, muttering or mumbling. Muttering or mumbling are included under this heading if actual words cannot be discerned. Music is a rare but well reported non-verbal hallucinatory experience.

One patient frequently heard 'the clicking noise of a computer'. There was no evidence of a delusion and it was concluded that he was experiencing a non-verbal auditory hallucination.

These phenomena are common in delirium and functional psychoses. Clinical experience is that they are common in early schizophrenia. As the disorder progresses there seems be a reduction of non-verbal auditory hallucinations and an increase in verbal auditory hallucinations.

Verbal auditory hallucinations

One or more voices may be heard. They may come from inside or outside the head. They may speak in unison, conduct a conversation between themselves, or address the patient. They are usually heard as speaking but they may be heard as singing. Voices rarely speak in complete sentences – they

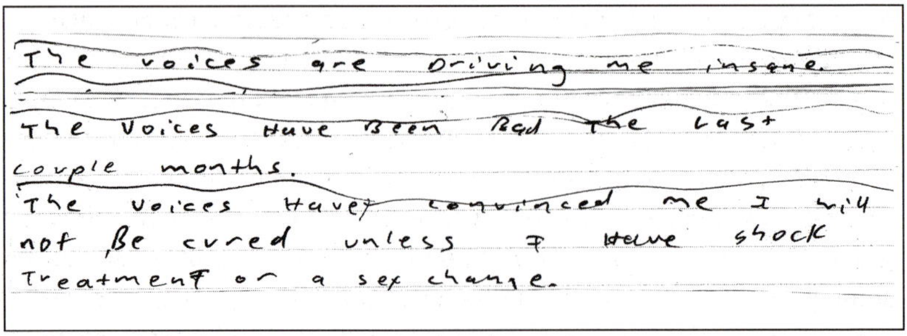

The voices are Driving me insane.

The Voices Have Been Bad the Last couple months.

The voices Have convinced me I will not Be cured unless I Have shock Treatment or a sex change.

Figure 34. These passages were written by a young man who suffered schizophrenia. A feature of his illness was auditory hallucinations, which he found to be unpleasant. (In contrast, some patients find auditory hallucinations to be pleasant or comforting.)

The third passage is a challenge. It is possible but unlikely that the voices told the patient that they would continue until he received electrical treatment or a sex change operation. It is also possible that this passage, which appears to be a disorder of the content of thought, may have arisen from a disorder of the form of thought. The hallucinations were distressing and relentless, suggesting that drastic measures would be necessary. Sexual ideation featured prominently in this man's thinking. That electrical treatment or a sex change operation would be helpful in alleviating 'the voices' could constitute illogical or derailed thinking.

usually say only a few disjointed words in a single utterance. While the content/meaning of the hallucinated words may have immediate meaning for the patient, more frequently they do not. Patients find great difficulty in repeating their auditory hallucinations verbatim. This is probably because hallucinations are generally reduced while the patient is in conversation and as many hallucinations make little sense, those heard earlier are difficult to remember (Figure 34).

An alert – the above comment about hallucinated voices being heard as short disjointed utterances extends to the situation where the hallucination is of two voices 'conversing' – that is, the voices do not conduct a sensible, extended conversation as one might hear on a crossed telephone line. Also, it very rarely happens that the patient can have a sustained conversation with hallucinated voices. What usually happens between a patient and hallucinations is a very brief 'yes it is – no it isn't' interchange.

Patient may recognise the voice as they have heard it before, either first hand or via the media. It may be that the patient has never heard the voice before, but believes he or she 'knows' to whom it belongs, even though the voice has made no statement on the matter. Patients may 'know' that an hallucinated voice is that of God, Jesus, the devil or a person about whom they had no former knowledge. Thus, such 'knowing' suggests the existence of a delusion.

The voice or voices may be heard speaking about the patient and therefore referring to the patient in the third person. They may comment on his or her thoughts or actions, or two or more voices may discuss the patient (meaning they make some brief poorly integrated comments).

Voices may instruct or command the patient to perform an act. Usually this is a trivial act such as making a cup of tea, but it may be to injure self or others. It is important for medicolegal and clinical reasons to know whether a patient complies with command hallucinations or not, and what are the consequences when she or he does not. When a command is first given, the voice is usually spoken, perhaps with a hint of insistence. For some patients, when command hallucinations are ignored, there are no consequences, the command is not repeated, or may be repeated essentially in the same manner, but they are able to continue with their original activities. In some cases, when commands are ignored they are repeated with much insistence, perhaps shouted and with terms of abuse attached. Generally, patients do not like complying with command hallucinations, perhaps because to do so weakens the sense of autonomy. However, it is very distressing to be subjected to the harassment of raised, abusive voices. A common response of patients is to comply with the trivial commands such as, 'look out of the window', and to resist the uncomfortable or dangerous ones such as, 'jump out of the window'. Command hallucinations are not a major factor in homicide compared to drunkenness or the important motive of jealousy. Almost without exception, patients find command hallucinations to injure themselves or others to be distressing. Should such hallucinations begin, most patients present for medical assistance.

Individuals who do not have command hallucinations sometimes claim to have them. These are generally individuals who wish to threaten others or to avoid responsibility for an act they have performed.

Dissociative hallucinations which arise in non-psychotic conditions are dealt with in a following section. Verbal auditory hallucinations of the type described above are most often features of organic disorders or conditions such as schizophrenia or psychotic mood disorder (severe depression of mania).

Dissociative hallucinations

The term 'dissociative' hallucination is not descriptive of the hallucination but suggests a general diagnostic area.

These hallucinations occur in non-psychotic individuals. This type of hallucination occur in two main circumstances – first, where the individual is a member of a subcultural group which sanctions such experiences – in these circumstances, the hallucination is usually in a religious or quasi-religious setting and the individual is in a dissociative state.

Second, dissociative hallucinations may occur where the individual does not belong to such a group. In these circumstance the hallucination occurs in a state of clear consciousness and motivating factors can be determined.

Unlike the 'verbal auditory hallucinations', those experiencing dissociative hallucinations can hold a conversation (a series of questions and answers) with the voice of a person, ghost or god. There may be associated visual, olfactory or tactile hallucinations.

Where this experience is sanctioned by the subculture to which the individual belongs, dissociative hallucinations may be regarded as a non-pathological hallucination. Where there is no such group membership, this experience is not usually a feature of psychosis and may be regarded as a dissociative phenomenon. It has been observed in suggestible histrionic personality, conversion disorder and factitious disorder. The presence of visual, olfactory or tactile hallucinations suggests that temporal lobe epilepsy should be excluded. Malingering is also to be considered

Mood-congruent and incongruent verbal hallucinations

Verbal hallucinations may be a feature of depressed or elevated mood. In the case of elevated mood the hallucination may assert the patient has exceptional beauty, intelligence or other qualities – 'Go to the palace, they will make you king' (Wing *et al.*, 1974). In the case of depressed mood the hallucinations may be denigratory or persecutory, or may suggest or command suicide.

A complication is that in acute, severe mood disorder, on rare occasions, hallucinations may occur which bear no apparent relationship to mood, such as, a voice commenting, 'She put on hat'. Such phenomena are recorded as auditory, verbal hallucinations – and as mood disorder is believed to be present it is worth adding the qualifier, 'mood incongruent'.

Hallucinations are a feature of severe mood disorder. They are not a feature of mild or moderate mood disorder and hallucinations suggesting suicide in a setting of mild mood disorder may be a dissociative phenomenon. If a person presents with hallucinations for the first time in middle life or later, even though they appear to have some depression which could explain matters, organic disorders such as space-occupying lesions must be excluded.

Tactile and somatic hallucinations

Tactile hallucinations are the experience of being touched or of something (almost invariably said to be insects) crawling under the skin (formication). These hallucinations are a feature of organic psychoses, particularly drug induced or withdrawal states. The sensation of being touched is a rare but possible feature of schizophrenia.

Somatic hallucinations are the sensation of things happening inside the body, such as organs moving from one part of the body to another. These are rare. They are often accompanied by delusional explanations and occur in schizophrenia.

Visual hallucinations

Visual hallucinations may be unformed (such as flashes of light) or formed (such as people). Figure 35, 36.

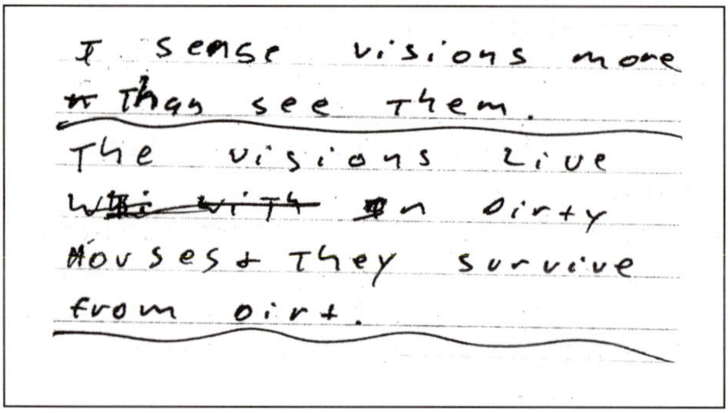

> I sense visions more
> ~~n~~ than see them.
> The visions live
> ~~with with~~ ~~on~~ on dirty
> houses & they survive
> from dirt.

Figure 35. These two passages were written by a young person who suffered schizophrenia.

It is unclear what he meant when he said he 'senses' visions. Some people experience straightforward visual hallucinations in which figures or objects are stationary or pass through their field of vision while they go about their daily tasks. Others report more difficult to categorize experiences (as here).

The second passage demonstrates how hallucinatory phenomena and delusionary material may combine to form even more complex psychopathology.

Given that this man lacked insight and was perplexed, frightened, and unresponsive to support, suicide was an ever-present concern.

Unformed hallucinations are usually of organic origin – ocular or central nervous system disorders. Formed hallucinations are also often of organic origin – upper brainstem or temporal cortex disorders.

Clinical experience is that a surprising number of patients with schizophrenia have visual hallucinations, sometimes of figures (either indistinct or detailed) standing to one side of the field of view. A recent study (Cutting, 1990) states that they occur in 15% of people with schizophrenia – it seems that we have not asked about them as much as they deserve.

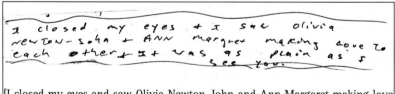

[I closed my eyes and saw Olivia Newton-John and Ann Margaret making love to each other & it was as plain as I see you]

Figure 36. This writing is from the same patient as in Figure 35 and the issue is again a phenomenon which sounds like visual hallucinations. Here he reports an experience which occurred when his eyes were closed which suggest the possibility of the voluntary imagination of scenes or delusional phenomena. However, he stated that he could 'see' these events 'as plain as I can see you' which increases the likelihood of this being a visual hallucination.

Gustatory and olfactory hallucinations

Hallucinations of taste and smell occur in organic disorders, most commonly in epilepsy.

Hallucinations of smell have been reported in schizophrenia – it is often difficult to distinguish from the delusion that one is being exposed (purposefully or non-purposefully) to toxic gases. It may also be necessary to differentiate from the somatic delusion that the patient is emitting a foul smell.

Alcoholic hallucinosis

Various types of hallucinations may occur in this condition, most commonly, auditory. They are often unpleasant – shouting abuse. This occurs in clear consciousness, distinct from the withdrawal state. Insight may be anywhere from absent to complete.

This condition occurs in individuals who have taken large amounts of alcohol over many years. Usually there has been recent cessation or marked reduction in consumption, but onset can occur during drinking bouts.

Illusions

Illusions are misperceptions of stimuli. They are usually transitory and can be corrected when attention is drawn to the mistake.

Illusions may occur in clouded consciousness, such as in delirium tremens, in which case objects such as creases in bed covers may be perceived as snakes, insects or other forms or animals. Illusions may also occur in aroused individuals without organic disorders or significant psychopathology, as in the case of a person walking in a dangerous location who misperceives a bush as a crouched attacker. Illusions appear to be very rare in non-organic psychiatric disorders.

7. Intelligence

The assessment of intelligence in the psychiatric examination is optional. The following paragraphs are offered for completeness.

Intelligence has proven so difficult to define that many have resorted to the non-definition, 'Intelligence is that which intelligence tests measure' (Reber, 1985). A useful definition was offered by Fish (Hamilton, 1974), 'the ability to think and act rationally and logically'.

Like some other functions found in this book, intelligence can be conceptualised (at least in part) not as a single entity but a composite of related entities. For example, Binet, the inventor of the intelligence test believed that intelligent behaviour depended on reasoning, imagination, insight, judgement and adaptability, and Rifkin (1991) casts the net even more broadly, 'Intellectual functioning includes memory, judgement, abstract thought, arithmetic calculations, and similar functions'.

While a definition has remained elusive, a range of intelligence tests has been developed. These are reliable and the capacities of individuals within a population fit the normal distribution curve. Where there is a need for a formal assessment of intelligence, a trained person should conduct a standardised test.

Intelligence tests were used to stratify people in educational and vocational settings for much of the twentieth century. The concept of intelligence continues to have theoretical and practical implications, but recently the suggestion has been made that intelligence has received unjustified importance while 'motivation' and/or 'will' have received insufficient emphasis, in attempts to predict capacity to perform and achieve in particular fields. The corollary is that people with very high intelligence test scores may still have personalities which render them unable to cooperate with others and thereby unable to achieve as expected.

In our own educational and vocational lives most of us have encountered people we consider to be more, and others we consider to be less, intelligent than ourselves. In daily life we make this judgement based on the speed at which people grasp what we are saying, their ability to have 'good ideas' and their ability to read, spell, debate and achieve high marks on scholastic and practical tests. The assessment of intelligence must rest on similar observations during interview and information from the personal history.

In examining the personal history for evidence of intelligence, particular attention is paid to scholastic achievement (relative to the energy expended), vocation and vocational success, and evidence of problem solving and good ideas. At interview, speed of thinking, ease with abstract concepts and verbal ability, the use of metaphor and particularly the vocabulary, will provide indicators. There should be a reasonable correlation between the indicators from the past and those of the present. Caution is necessary.

Authorities have described retardation and dementia in terms of the failure to develop, or the loss of, intellectual functions (Reber, 1985). Recently, however, these diagnostic criteria have been extended. DSM-IV mental retardation includes, in addition to significantly subaverage general intellectual functioning, significant limitations in adaptive functions (which are skills such as communication, self-care and work), while DSM-IV dementia includes memory impairments and at least one other cognitive deficit (such as apraxia, aphasia and agnosia). Thus, the term intelligence has been largely replaced with the no more precise but broader term, cognition. (See related entries on Cognition and The Frontal Lobes.)

If the intellectual capacity is assessed at interview as being less than expected from the history, it is necessary to consider the possibility of a dementing disorder (such as Alzheimer's disease), brain trauma or other intracranial pathology, or a general medical condition (such as hypothyroidism). Research has demonstrated reduced intelligence test performance in those suffering schizophrenia and major depressive disorder. The clinician must remain aware that mistakes are easily made.

If the intellectual capacity is assessed at interview as being greater than expected, exclude the possibility that the patient is mildly hypomanic, taking stimulants or exercising engaging personality skill.

8. Cognition

In psychology, the term 'cognition' has been used to mean thinking and the mental processes of knowing and becoming aware. Thus, it has been used to cover some of the areas already considered in this book (such as thinking). In neurology and psychiatry, cognition has been used to mean the same as 'higher cortical functions', which includes memory, orientation, concentration, language (examined by tests of speaking, reading and writing) recognition of stimuli (examined by tests for agnosia) and performance of learned skilled movements (examined by tests for apraxia). Some neurologists also include mood, personality and other mental state phenomena under the heading of higher cortical functions but psychiatrists do not endorse those inclusions.

Tests are used to detect the presence of certain disorders. Formerly, tests of cognition were used to identify the 'organic' disorders, but this term is becoming less precise and the examiner needs to be aware of some subtleties. The label organic was coined at a time when investigative technologies were crude. It was assumed that if no organic basis could be demonstrated with the technology of the day, none existed. The conditions excluded by this process were termed 'functional'. Genetics and imaging studies are now demonstrating the organic basis of many of what were called the functional disorders.

Cognitive testing is valuable in detecting some conditions which may present as psychiatric disorders but which require the services of other branches of medicine, for example, patients may present with a picture suggestive of schizophrenia or depression which is secondary to space-occupying lesions, toxic, endocrine or metabolic abnormalities. In such circumstances, cognitive testing is likely to reveal inconsistent deficits and indicate the need for further investigation and medical or surgical treatment.

Cognitive testing may unequivocally indicate that an organic condition is present, for example, a young bank manager who is able to learn new material at one interview but not at another. Most often the exact nature of the disorder will require special investigations. Often, consultation with another medical specialist will be necessary. Neuropsychological testing can confirm and extend knowledge of the cognitive deficits; it should not be used to establish that which can be established by the psychiatric examination.

It may not be appropriate or necessary to perform all the cognitive testing at the first interview. Cognitive testing involves a lot of questions. These may be construed as a threatening interrogation or an irritating, irrelevant waste of time. For example, in the case of a woman who presents with distress arising from domestic violence and who expects to be made a 'scapegoat', it is better for the male examiner to note that the delivery of the history and mental state examination suggest the patient is orientated and able to remember, concentrate and use language effectively, and for formal cognitive testing to be delayed (it may not need to be performed).

In general, if memory, orientation, concentration and language are intact, recognition and performance of learned skilled movements will also be intact. Thus, the former may be regarded as a screening test for the latter, such that if the former is intact, the latter need not be tested. This system is not without risk as exceptions may occur and caution is necessary. However, it is economical of clinical time and is recommended.

The examiner should be capable of exploring the cognitive functions using a variety of tests and techniques. Frequently a patient is encountered who has already been assessed by others using the standard methods – this introduces the complication of learning effect and it may be necessary to go beyond the standard methods. Also, frequently, patient responses are equivocal, again raising the need for additional skills.

The Mini-Mental State Examination (MMSE) (Folstein *et al.*, 1975) deserves special mention. This is a standardised, internationally accepted screening test of cognitive functions which is used by a wide range of medical and paramedical professionals. It examines orientation in some detail and then briefly touches on registration and recall, attention and concentration, language and constructional abilities. Brevity is its strength (allowing a wide breadth examination) and its weakness (not allowing in depth examination). Because of the learning effect it should not be repeatedly administered. Well administered, the MMSE gives a very valuable quantification of the cognitive functions. If this screening test indicates reason for concern, more extensive testing should be conducted. The ability to administer the MMSE should not be regarded as sufficient cognitive testing skill for the psychiatric examiner.

A 'catastrophic reaction' may occur when the cognitively impaired individual becomes aware of his or her deficits. This usually takes the form of sudden emotional distress, often with an angry outbursts or crying. It may be triggered by the challenge thrown up by the normal events of life, such as failure in operating a complicated television set, which the patient has formerly been able to operate. It may also occur clinically when testing is pursued relentlessly, in spite of the patient's demonstrated failure. This may be unavoidable in some circumstances. In ordinary clinical practice, however, it is sufficient to ask questions which the patient can answer, move on to more difficult material, and if the patient fails and gives any indication of annoyance or frustration, finish by returning to the level at which he or she is competent. This may be illustrated with an example from the testing of orientation in time. If, from the history and introductory conversation, it is assessed that the patient has some impairment, a reasonable question would be to ask the patient to name the month. If successfully answered, it is appropriate to ask for the day of the week. If the patient fails to answer this correctly, it is better not to go directly on to the date, but to then ask for the year. If the year is not successfully given, there are clearly problems with orientation in time. If the year is successfully answered, to confirm the earlier impression given by the failure with the day, it is now possible (after the recent success with the year) to go on to ask the day of the week again and the date.

Memory

Memory is the ability to revive past thoughts and sensory experiences. It includes three basic mental processes: registration (the ability to perceive, recognise and establish information in the central nervous system), retention (the ability to retain registered information) and recall (the ability to retrieve stored information at will).

Psychological and biological data support the existence of a short-term memory store (STS) and a long-term memory store (LTS). The STS has limited capacity and holds information for brief periods. To learn information for longer periods, it must be transferred to the LTS, a system of essentially unlimited capacity, which can hold information indefinitely.

Short-term memory (which for this discussion includes what has been called immediate memory by others) has been defined as the reproduction, recognition or recall of perceived material within a period of up to 30 seconds after presentation. For testing purposes, long-term memory can be split into two extremes: recent memory (events occurring during the past few hours or days); and remote (events occurring in past years).

There is discussion about whether short-term memory meets all the definitional criteria of memory – that is, in short-term tests the information is held in a manner which does not require the same process of recall as is required for long-term memory. This matter cannot be resolved here, but the relationship between STS and LTS will prove to be important.

The classification of memory and related topics is problematic – the structure provided is not perfect and there is some redundancy.

Tests of memory

During the psychiatric interview some information about memory will be available from the history and conversation of the patient. Memory tests are required for quantitative assessment. Three levels of memory are specifically tested.

The examiner is conducting a professional examination and should proceed confidently. There should be concern for the patient's comfort and dignity, but these will not be offended by an examiner who proceeds in a courteous, professional manner. There should not be indecision or inappropriate apology. Cognitive testing is better commenced after at least some more general conversation. The examiner should then say something like, 'Thank you Mr X, I understand what you have been saying. I now need to test your memory'. Then proceed directly to, 'I am going to give you three things which I want you to remember...' or similar words, depending on the test the examiner wishes to apply.

In practice, it is only a narrow band of mildly to moderately impaired individuals who find testing threatening and may object. The completely intact individual will understand the importance of the procedure and will not object if treated respectfully. Nor will the severely impaired individual who does not have insight into his or her poor test performance. When a patient who has been treated respectfully refuses memory, or other cognitive testing, there is probably cognitive impairment.

History and conversation

Memory can be influenced by many factors. In addition to organic lesions, intoxication (the only indicator of which may be the smell of an intoxicant), inability to attend, emotional arousal, psychomotor retardation, thought disorder and motivation must be considered.

Patients should be able to give a clear account of their life from the remote to the recent past. Quite often, the examiner will have no information against which to test the patient's account, but useful indicators can be gained, nevertheless.

The presenting complaint is important. Where memory function is of primary concern the patient may not be able to remember why she or he is present or may offer poor memory as the reason for the presentation. Full details of any claimed memory loss and the associated affect displayed at that time are investigated and recorded. It may be necessary to distinguish loss of memory from loss of insight. Irrespective of insight, the patient should be able to give an account of the events of the days before and the day of the interview. For example, the patient should be able to give details of who made the arrangements for the interview, how the patient was conveyed from home or work, at what time did the patient depart home or work, time of arrival and how long the journey took. Thus, the history gives the opportunity for a real-life test of the recent memory.

Assessment of the remote memory may prove difficult. The examiner usually has no information against which to check the patient's account, and with some conditions (Alzheimer's disease for example) the patient may hide and deny memory difficulties. The internal consistency of the history, especially in the relating of the personal history, may give important indications. This is the matching of dates, ages and events when the patient is describing different aspects of past life. The names and current ages of children and siblings are often useful. Inconsistencies indicate difficulties with remote memory.

Short-term (immediate) memory test

The most common test is to ask the patient to repeat sequences of digits. Three digits are given first and the patient is asked to repeat them. If this is performed successfully, four digits are given and so on, until the patient makes mistakes. A normal person of average intelligence is usually able to repeat seven digits correctly. When mistakes begin, it is usual for the patient to be able to recall the first and the last digits. It is believed that the last are recalled because they remain in the STS, the first are recalled because they have been transferred into the LTS, and the middle digits are lost as they have been displaced from the STS by the last digits.

Another test is the ability to reverse digits. This is not recommended. There is no agreement on how many digits the normal individual is able to reverse, and it appears to depend more strongly than the forward digit test on the ability to concentrate.

Recent memory test

Recent memory is the most recently formed long-term memory. The ability to create new long-term memories is essential for independent living.

An essential feature of tests is that after the test material is presented, other material is presented so that the test material is displaced from the STS.

A common method is to test the patient's ability to learn three or four unrelated words. Patients are advised that their memory should be tested, that they will be given some words to remember, and that later in the interview they will be asked to recall them. The words are said at the rate of about one word per second. The patient is asked to repeat them, to ensure that they have been registered properly. The interview then proceeds and the patient is distracted and must attend to other material. Some minutes later the patient is asked to recall the words.

Some authors require patient to remember three and others four words. In either case, the patient is expected to recall all words accurately.

Other tests include giving the patient a name and address or a short story to remember.

Remote memory test

The examiner usually does not have extensive knowledge of the patient's early life against which to compare answers to questions. Individual differences in intelligence and education make it difficult to know what questions on past world events it would be reasonable to ask.

The date of birth is often available to the examiner. However, this is very highly learned material, it is among the last pieces of information to be lost and its retention does not exclude moderately advanced memory problems.

The names and dates of birth of the patient's children may also be available, as might the patient's wife's (in the case of a married male) and mother's maiden name, and these form reasonable questions.

It is reasonable to ask the capital cities of Australia, England and USA, and the dates of the first and second world wars – taking care to take account of intelligence and education.

Another method is to ask the patient to name ten colours, ten animals, ten fruit and ten capital cities. The production of less than twenty items, in total, strongly suggests memory problems.

Loss of memory/amnesia – clinical pictures

Loss of memory of organic origin

Dementia

Dementia is a global deterioration in intellectual functioning, a central feature of which is loss of memory. It is usually of gradual onset, although it may follow sudden events such as head injury. In general, the more recently stored memories are lost first, and those stored long ago are lost last. However, this is a relative matter and the remote memory of patients with dementia is usually significantly impaired compared with that of non-demented persons of comparable age. There is also impairment in abstract thinking, judgement, other cortical functions and personality change.

In the psychiatric interview, when dementia is considered, attention is paid to short-term and recent memory. Of these, special attention is paid to the assessment of recent memory, partly because this is technically easy, and partly because recent memory is evidence of the ability to form new long-term memories.

A wide range of diseases may reult in dementia. The most common are the parenchymatous diseases of the brain, of which the most common is Alzheimer's disease. Others include Pick's disease and Huntington's disease. Vascular disease is a common cause. Multiple sclerosis and Parkinson's disease may also cause dementia, but in such conditions, any dementia may be overshadowed by the physical signs of the disease. Infection is becoming an important cause because of HIV-related disorders; other infections include Creutzfeldt-Jacob disease, viral encephalitis, cryptococcal meningitis, neurosyphilis, cerebral tuberculosis and fungal meningitis. Metabolic diseases, deficiency states and drugs also need to be considered.

Amnestic disorder (Korsakoff's psychosis/syndrome)

The amnestic disorder is characterised by memory loss (particularly recent and of short-term memory, and to a lesser extent, remote memory). The important test is for recent memory – the formation of new long-term memory is the major problem. In contrast to dementia, the other cognitive functions and the personality are relatively unimpaired. Lack of motivation and flat affect are common. Patients frequently lack insight or deny difficulties. Confabulation may occur in the early stages, but usually disappears over time.

Confabulation is a curious phenomenon. It occurs when a patient has no memory for a certain period or event and when asked about it, gives an account which (of course) is completely inaccurate. It is particularly interesting when the account is unbelievable – such as, 'yesterday I flew a plane to the North Pole to check on the penguins'. Confabulation does not always involve unbelievable events and the accounts become more mundane as the amnestic disorder abates. One definition states that confabulation involves 'untrue experiences which the patient believes'. Caution is required. Patients believe these accounts so for them, the accounts are true and they may recount these so-called 'untrue' events with conviction and arousal. Cases have been reported in which the confabulated details are always the same (in spite of memory loss) but in many cases these change with each examination. While there is much variation in the clinical presentation of this phenomenon, the term should be reserved for use when the 'untrue experiences' fill a hole in the memory – it should not used synonymously with the term delusion.

The most common cause of amnestic disorder is thiamine deficiency secondary to alcohol use – in which case onset may be gradual, or more apparently rapid if it arises out of an acute Wernicke's encephalopathy. Head injury, cerebral neoplasm, carbon monoxide poisoning and herpes simplex encephalitis are other causes.

Loss of memory of psychological origin

Psychogenic amnesia

In psychogenic amnesia the predominant disturbance is an episode of inability to recall important personal information, which is not due to an organic mental disorder. Onset is sudden (except in the case of multiple personality [dissociative identity disorder]) and there is usually some precipitating emotional trauma. The psychogenic amnesias are reversible.

Although discrete types are listed, the usual picture is a mixture of two or more. The clinical presentation is compounded by the combination of unconscious forgetting and active avoidance of painful material. Malingering must be excluded. The memory and the understanding of the patient of his or her condition will vary with time and circumstances.

Several types have been described:
· **Localised** – loss of memory for a short period of time
· **Generalised** – loss of memory for the whole of life
· **Selective** – failure to recall some but not all events during a short period of time
· **Continuous** – forgetting each successive event as it occurs.

Psychogenic fugue

This is a rare condition in which there is unexpected travel away from the customary domicile, with inability to recall the past.

Multiple personality disorder

In this disorder there exists within the person, two or more distinct personalities, each with their own patterns of perceiving relating to and thinking about the environment. One is often unaware of another and there may be no memory of the experience of one by another.

Paramnesia

Paramnesia is a term that does not have wide usage, but is useful in psychiatry as a box into which certain phenomena, such as *déjà vu*, can be placed. A formal definition states that paramnesia is 'the falsification of memory by distortion of recall'. This 'falsification' occurs without any purposeful intention to deceive.

The term is derived from the Greek, *para* meaning 'irregular' and *mnesia* meaning 'memory' – hence, 'a distorted or false memory'.

Alternatively, paramnesias have been included under the dissociative disorders (West, 1976), in which case the importance of accompanying feeling is emphasised – 'distortions of memory which are often accompanied by strange feelings of such intensity that they could be considered hallucinations of sensibilities'.

Confabulation

Confabulation has been defined as the unconscious filling of gaps in memory by imaginary or untrue experiences that the patient believes, but which has no basis in fact. It has been discussed under Amnestic disorder, and the reader is encouraged to consult that entry.

Depersonalisation and derealisation

Depersonalisation is described as an alteration in the perception or experience of the self, and derealisation is an alteration in the perception of one's surroundings such that the reality of the external world is lost. These are dealt with in more detail under the heading of Perception.

Déjà vu *and* Jamais vu

Déjà vu is the false feeling of visual recognition in which a new situation is incorrectly regarded as a repetition of a previous memory.

Jamais vu is the false feeling of unfamiliarity with a real situation one has experienced.

Déjà vu and *Jamais vu* are not important mental state phenomena. Both are experienced from time to time by individuals without significant psychopathology. It is possible that they are experienced more commonly by patients with significant psychopathology but there is no evidence one way or the other.

Reduplicative phenomena

Patients may have the experience that they have been duplicated and are in two different places at the same time, or that the place they are in or other people around them have been duplicated. These conditions are difficult to distinguish from other memory and perceptual, non-psychotic and psychotic disorders.

The experience of being in two places at the same time is similar to out of body experiences described by individuals without serious psychopathology. The experience that places have been duplicated has been observed following head injury. Capgra's syndrome is the experience that a person quite close to the patient has been replaced by a double – this is a psychotic disorder, most often seen in schizophrenia.

Orientation

Orientation in the psychiatric examination means the state of awareness of one's relationships and surroundings in terms of time, place and person. Insofar as disorientated people are frequently given orienting information by other individuals, but remain disorientated, the condition has a memory component. Other important influences may be apraxia, agnosia and attentional difficulties.

The patient will accept a memory test without discomfort or distress when it is presented as a required part of a routine examination. Tests of orientation may cause a little distress in the patient and apprehension in the examiner, as they imply not merely that the memory may be impaired, but that the patient may not even know where he or she is in time and space. Here are three tips.

1) After testing memory, proceed, perhaps after some more general conversation (a rest from testing), to test orientation as an extension of the testing format already established. It may be appropriate to say, 'Yes I see, thank you. I would like now to test you a little further...'.
2) Spend time establishing rapport with the patient before testing is applied. This will allow the examiner to obtain cues about the level of function and the level at which to pitch.

3) It is better to first ask questions that are close to the level of the patient's ability. If the patient appears to be functioning normally, it may be appropriate to first ask if he or she can give the date and the floor/level of the building where the examination is being conducted, rather than the year or the city. Where there is uncertainty, it may be easier to ask for the month and the name of the building first. If these are answered incorrectly, proceed to the bigger picture questions – if answered correctly, return to the fine grain questions.

Orientation in time

Orientation in time is the first dimension to be lost and the last to return. The patient is asked to give the year, month, day of the week and date. As with memory, it is the recent, more precise information which is lost first. It is often argued that patients in hospital have no need to be aware of, and few cues as to, the day of the week and the date. This needs to be taken into account, but the cognitively normal patient will, on most occasions, give the correct day of the week. This is particularly important if the patient is being interviewed at a clinic or ward round which is held on a weekday (which are busy days when the senior staff attend) and in response to the question, gives a weekend day (which are less busy days when the senior staff do not attend).

Even more recent and precise information is the time of day, and the same objections about the lack of cues do not apply, as patients take meals, and have access to clocks and the usual indicators. Objections can continue that patients do not have the same need to know the time as they have little to do, but the facts are that cognitively normal people are not content not to think and are able to give an accurate account of the time of day. Clinical experience is that disorientated patients often give answers that are inconsistent with the evidence. They may contend it is evening even when the sun is blazing through the window, and may not change their claim when this inconsistency is pointed out. When trying to help the patient with the time of day the examiner may ask which meals of the day the patient has eaten. This is a test of memory, but can be used this way in testing orientation – the disorientated patient may claim that it is late afternoon, but that breakfast has not yet been taken.

Orientation in place

The Mini-Mental State Exam (Folstein *et al.,* 1975) contains some good questions on this topic. At the 'big picture' end, the questions are about identifying the city and the county. This may not be analogous to asking about the month and the year. It may be that the patient loses the month before the year, but the state before the city – work on this point has not been reported. If a patient knows the city, then knowing the county is a matter of memory, rather than orientation. This is a further example of the indistinct boundary between orientation and memory.

A reasonable place to start testing orientation in place is with the city or the building. Going on from other questions the examiner can say something like, 'Well, thank you for answering those questions, Mrs Z. Now, I would like to ask you, can you please tell me, the name of the city (or building) we are now in?' It is important to get the precise name of the building. If it is a small hospital or nursing home some distance from the patient's usual domicile, a generalisation such as 'Hospital' may be acceptable. In the case of a well known facility close to the usual domicile, the exact or almost exact name can be expected. In either circumstance, it is reasonable to ask the patient, 'Yes, you are quite right, this is a hospital. But, can you please tell me which hospital it is?'.

If the patient is not able to give the name of the building, or gives an incorrect answer it is important to determine whether they can benefit from the cues around them. If they answer that they are in their own home, it is reasonable to say something like, 'I'm not sure this is your house. Is this your furniture? There seem to be other people walking around. Are you sure this is your home?'.

For patients who say they do not know where they are, the same sort of questions as in the above paragraph should be asked. It is reasonable to say something like, 'Mr Y, we are in a public building. It could be a police station, a railway station, a fire station or a hospital. Have a look around. Look at the beds and the people walking around. In which one of those places do you think we are?'.

If patients answer incorrectly or are unable to give an answer to the name of the building, it is recommended that they be taken to a window and asked to identify any local landmarks or prominent buildings. They should then be asked if this helps them in working out their present location – 'Yes, Ms D, that is the Police Station across the road, and that is Liverpool Street. So, where are we then? What is in Liverpool Street, across the road from the Police Station?'.

Patients who give the name of the facility/hospital correctly, should then be asked to name the ward. If this cannot be given, the patient should be asked what type of cases are treated on this ward. If there are difficulties with this question, ask the patient to look around, 'You are right about this being the ward of the City Hospital. But, what type of ward is this?

Have a look around – the patients don't seem to be in bed here. Do you think this is a surgical ward where people are recovering from operations?'.

The answer to the question of what sort of ward the patient has been admitted to can be useful. Patients who lacks insight into their disorder and do not know the nature of the ward to which they have been admitted are likely to be suffering form cognitive loss, which usually means an organic disorder. Patients who lack insight into their disorder but know the nature of the ward to which they have been admitted may be suffering a functional disorder. This is a generalisation and there are exceptions. (Not all organic conditions have associated cognitive loss and functional disorders can be so severe that the patient is unable to communicate an awareness of surroundings.)

Orientation in person

Orientation in person requires various abilities, including the capacity to recognise faces (prosopagnosia being agnosia for faces) and memory. Thus, failure in orientation in person is a general rather than specific indicator of pathology.

Under this heading the examiner is to assess patients' ability to identify not only themselves, but others. A common mistake is to report only the patient's ability to give his or her own name. This is over-learned information and one of the last pieces to be lost. Perhaps of more importance is the patient's ability to identify others. In the history there may be accounts of the patient not recognising his or her children (this is quite common and a source of distress to the children of patients suffering from progressive dementing disorders).

Orientation in person may be tested by asking patients to identify themselves. The patient may then asked to identify the examiner, who will have introduced himself or herself earlier (and may have been known from previous meetings) and to indicate the type of work in which the examiner is engaged. Patients may say that they have a poor head for names. It is a test of memory to give the examiner's name again and re-test later. From the point of view of orientation it is better to move to the examiners function, by saying something like, 'Yes, I'm not much good on names myself. But we've been talking about different things for a few minutes, Mr X ... Can you tell me what sort of work I do?' This is a good, broad test of cognitive function.

When testing orientation in person it is often better to ask the patient to identify by name and occupation, any available nursing staff who have had dealing with the patient, and any available relatives. If any of the patient's children are available, they should be brought into the office and the patient should be asked to give the offspring's dates of birth and position in the sibship. The patient may be asked to give the name of the spouse and the names of any children born to available relatives.

Attention (concentration)

The term concentration does not appear in dictionaries of psychology and is often absent from the indexes of psychiatric textbooks. It has been used interchangeably with attention. Simple definitions include that attention is the ability to focus on the matter at hand and that concentration is the ability to sustain that focus. While this distinction makes sense, it is not widely held. Perhaps through tradition, concentration still appears in some accounts of mental state assessment – but in the present account the preferred term is attention.

Attention is a multifaceted mental function, but in general, it denotes the capacity of an individual to focus the mind on some aspect of the environment or the contents of the mind itself (Cutting, 1992).

Attention is understood in the context of consciousness. Consciousness is a state of awareness of the self and the environment. The experience of consciousness depends on attention, which can be approached from three aspects: intensity, selectivity and voluntary effort. Intensity (tonic or basal arousal or activation) is a non-specific process, which prepares the organism to meet the challenges of the environment and depends on the action of the reticular formation. Selectivity of attention brings certain aspects of the environment into focus. This may be both voluntary and involuntary. With voluntary selectivity, extraneous signals are suppressed, while with involuntary selectivity there is the startle or orienting response (when the organism meets a new stimuli) and the habituation response (the gradual diminution of responses to continued or repeated stimuli). Voluntary effort is also required, and this is believed to depend, in large part, on fully functional frontal lobes (Horvath, 1991).

Disorders of attention

The disorder of attention can be classified as subtle or severe. This is a crude classification – there is no quantification and categorisation depends on experience and opinion.

Subtle disorder of attention

Many of the severe forms of the so-called functional psychiatric disorders (depressive psychosis, mania, anxiety and schizophrenia) and some of the less severe organic disorders (delirium, dementia and brain injury) show subtle disorders of attention.

Severe disorder of attention

Some of the most severe cases of the so-called functional psychiatric disorders (especially the most severe cases of schizophrenia and depressive psychosis) and most cases of delirium, dementia and brain damage show severe disorder of attention.

Tests of attention

Rather than enter into a complicated explanation about the nature of attention and the need for yet anther type of examination, it is better for the examiner to continue on from the testing of memory without emphasising the change in focus.

It must be borne in mind that the arousal stimulated by the examination process may make the task of attending very difficult.

History and conversation

Patients often lack insight into their difficulties with attention. However, insight may be present, especially where there is functional psychiatric disorder (depression, anxiety and schizophrenia) and the experience and the knowledge is often unpleasant. Patients are more often familiar with the word concentration, thus in talking with them, this word is recommended. Where the symptom is not complained of but is suspected (by the examiner), it is reasonable to ask, 'Mr X, how is your concentration at the moment. Are you able to watch a show on TV and concentrate all the way through?'. Alternatively, it may be more appropriate to ask particular patients whether they are able to concentrate on reading the newspaper.

There may be other symptoms which make it difficult for the patient to attend to tasks, such as distraction by hallucinations and delusions and loss of interest. These need to be considered. There may be occasions when there is little distraction and the patient has at least some interest, but the ability to concentrate is still subjectively impaired. Examples include moderate to severe depression where the patient complains bitterly about the inability to concentrate on the written word – even with concerted effort the patient may be unable to concentrate and extract meaning from a paragraph of the newspaper.

Where there are marked difficulties with attention, this will be obvious during conversation. The patient will be unable to give a clear account of the reasons for presentation, will wander off the topic and will be distracted by the external environment and thoughts. It may be difficult, initially, to distinguish the person with delirium from the person with schizophrenia and severe formal thought disorder.

Subtraction

A common test is to ask the patient to take seven from one hundred and keep subtracting seven from the answer. It is frequently stated that the time taken and the number of mistakes should be recorded, but there is no accepted limit on the number of mistakes and the amount of time allowed. As with other cognitive tasks, a written record of the performance may have value if the ability is re-tested at another time. Even without strict rules, it is often possible to identify impaired ability. The patient may not even perform the first subtraction correctly. Often an impaired patient will subtract a number of times (with mistakes), then make some additions (of various amounts) and finally get lost and stop.

It is always necessary to take into account that the arousal of the testing situation may detract from the performance. If the patient is of lower intelligence or has had little numerical education, it may be appropriate to give an easier task. Subtracting three from twenty down to zero is easier. Subtracting two from twenty is easier again. Finally, for certain individuals, a reasonable numerical task is to count back from twenty to zero, one at a time. It is important only that the task taxes the patient so that his or her ability to attend and to sustain attention can be evaluated.

Reversing components

Reversing a series of numbers is a commonly suggested test. The examiner reads the numbers to the patient slowly and clearly. It is not clear what constitutes normal and pathological performances.

Reversing the letters of a word is stated to be an alternative to the 100 minus 7 test in the MMSE (Folstein *et al.*, 1975) for the non-numerically trained person. This is quite a reasonable test, but would be just as well to ask patients to perform the reversal of a series of numbers – in the reversing numbers test the patient is not asked to perform any numerical task, simply to rearrange the order of the symbols. Perhaps it could be claimed that to the numerically naive individual, being faced with a task involving numbers may be especially arousing and unnecessarily detract from the performance.

When testing the ability to spell a word backwards, the patient should be comfortable with the forward arrangement of the letters, so the examiner should first say the word, then spell it forward slowly – then, finally, ask the patient to reverse the letters.

Reversing the months of the year is another recommended test. The problems with this test are that some people learn this task as a rote skill at school and others do not – for those without this learning, reversing the months of the year is quite a difficult exercise. An easier and appropriate task for the less intellectually gifted is to reverse the days of the week. The problem may be that this task is too easy – it can be made more difficult by asking the patient to reverse the days of the week for a fortnight. As stated above, what is being tested is not the patient's ability to produce the correct answer but the patient's ability to attend, and the examiner may have to make a decision based on a combination of tests that are too difficult and too easy.

Other cognitive (higher cortical) functions

The combination of a thorough psychiatric and physical examination (which includes a neurological examination) enables the confident diagnosis of psychiatric disorders. With these skills the psychiatrist will also be able to make some neurological diagnoses and identify those cases in which the opinion of other experts (neurologist, neuropsychiatrist, neuropsychologist, speech pathologist) are required.

The following cognitive tests are appropriate in certain neuropsychiatric disorders.

Language

This is an area where psychiatric and neurological classifications duplicate and overlap to some extent. This in part arises out of the different history of the disciplines and the unsatisfactory division of disorders into functional and organic categories.

In the psychiatric examination, with attention focused on the functional disorders, utterances which did not obey the usual rules were often classified as disorders of the form of thought. In the neurological examination, with attention focused on the organic disorders, similar utterances are included under the current heading (language).

An outline of some neurological disorders and terminology gives a context for the tests of language.

Aphasia

Aphasia is defined as the loss or impairment of language caused by brain damage (Benson, 1992). Two important points immediately emerge. First, as aphasia includes 'impairment' it is not necessary to introduce the additional term dysphasia (meaning dysfunction of speech). Second, there is specific mention that this problem is the result of 'brain damage' – purposefully and traditionally, excluding the application of this term from use in the so-called functional disorders.

Paraphasia is the production of unintentional syllables, words, or phrases during speech. However, paraphasia has also been defined as 'partial aphasia' (Dorland, 1914) thereby indicating a link with brain damage. Were it not for this link with brain damage, paraphasia could be used interchangeably with formal thought disorder, for that symptom undeniably manifests 'unintentional syllables, words or phrases'. When utterances are transcribed onto paper, it is impossible to determine with certainty which are better classified as the examples of 'disorders of the form of thought' and which are better classified as 'a paraphasia'. That is not to claim that these are the same phenomena with the same pathophysiology.

Types of aphasia

Broca's aphasia

In Broca's aphasia the output is sparse, effortful, dysarthric, dysprosodic, short-phrased and agrammatical. There is disturbance in repetition and naming. Comprehension is relatively preserved. The patient may be aware of, and frustrated by, the expressive difficulties. This form is associated with dominant frontal opercular involvement.

Wernicke's aphasia

In Wernicke's aphasia there is fluent verbal output with normal word count and phrase length and no effort or articulatory problems, but there is difficulty in word finding and frequent paraphasic substitution. There is striking disturbance of comprehension. Difficulty with repeating reflects the disturbance of comprehension. The patient may be unaware of these difficulties and frustrated by the failure of others to respond appropriately. This form is associated with lesions of the posterior superior temporal lobe of the dominant hemisphere.

Conduction aphasia

In conduction aphasia there is fluent verbal output and good ability to comprehend, but severe disturbance in repetition. Paraphasias are common. Writing is often abnormal. This form is frequently associated with lesions of the supramarginal gyrus.

Transcortical aphasia

The striking feature of transcortical aphasia is the preservation of repeating in the presence of marked language impairment. There are sensory and motor forms of transcortical aphasia.

Nominal aphasia

In nominal aphasia the primary problem is with word finding. There are frequent pauses and a stumbling output. There may be reading and writing disturbance. Output may be fluent and comprehension good, but naming is significantly disturbed. This form commonly follows recovery from other types of aphasia.

Dysarthria

Dysarthria (speech disorder due to organic disorders of the speech organs or nervous system) is a mechanical problem. Aphasia is a disorder of the symbolic functions of speech. Dysarthria may coexist with aphasia, as in Broca's aphasia, or alone, as in cerebellar damage or bulbar palsy. While dysarthria is not a form of aphasia, it is convenient to include it here.

Testing aphasia

Observations are made during introductory conversation and while the history is being given. If the possibility of an organic disorder is raised, additional testing is appropriate. The following abilities may be tested.

Mechanics of speech

This is, in fact, a test of dysarthria, but the mechanism of speech must be checked before the examination of the ability to communicate meaning by speech. The patient is asked to produce the vowel 'ah' steadily for as long as possible, and to produce a sting of consonants ('puh-puh-puh...'). Tongue twisters may also be used. Any tongue twister will do, traditionally popular have been, 'West Register Street', and 'Around the rugged rocks, the ragged rascals ran'.

Fluency, phrase length and paraphasic substitutions

At this level there is no specific test for these features. They are observed throughout the examination and notes are kept.

Comprehension

When it is necessary to test comprehension, the examiner must be alert to the possibility that apraxia and agnosia may be complicating the case. The patient may be asked: 'Close your eyes', and be given some information such as a short story and asked to repeat it in his or her own words. Comprehension should be tested both verbally and in writing (mentioned again later).

Repetition

The patient is asked to repeat verbatim, short passages of normal speech.

Naming

The patient is asked to name objects on the examiner's person or around the room, such as, watch, tie, pencil, pillow and chair.

Writing ability

The patient is given writing equipment and asked to write a sentence. The patient's educational background must be taken into account. The patient may be embarrassed and claim not to be able to think of anything to write. In such circumstances the examiner can dictate a short sentence, or the patient can be asked to write his or her name and address (the examiner being alert that such help alters the 'Write a sentence' test).

Reading ability

The patient is asked to read a passage aloud. Note is taken not only of how well this task is performed, but also whether what was read was comprehended and could be acted upon – such as the MMSE written instruction 'Close your eyes'.

Diagnostic implications of aphasia

Severe aphasia with many paraphasias may be difficult to distinguish from schizophrenic thought with marked disorder of form. On very rare occasions it may be impossible to distinguish between them, so the symptom is ignored and a diagnosis is made using the remaining signs and symptoms.

Aphasia is, by definition, a symptom of organic disorder – the most common being vascular and space-occupying lesions. When aphasia is being considered, a full neurological examination is mandatory. As small lesions may be otherwise silent, special investigations including imaging can be useful.

Other language disorders

The following conditions are rare. They are included here for the sake of completeness and because of they indicate the frailty of the functional-organic distinction.

Amelodia (affective motor aprosodia)

Amelodia is characterised by flat, monotonous verbal output, decreased facial movement, and reduced use of gesture (Benson, 1992). It can be tested by having the patient hum a familiar tune such as Happy Birthday, a nursery rhyme, or the national anthem.

It has been described as the result of pathology (usually cerebrovascular accident) of the right frontal opercular area. However, depressive disorder and schizophrenia have similar symptoms and need to be seriously considered.

Verbal dysdecorum

In contrast to the above examples, in verbal dysdecorum, language is not defective. There is loss of control of the contents of verbal output. The patient speaks too freely, discusses improper topics, argues and is 'otherwise disagreeable' (Benson, 1992). There may or may not be physical impropriety.

It has been described as the result of right frontal pathology. However, hypomania has similar symptoms and would need to be seriously considered.

Skilled movement and apraxia

Apraxia is a disorder of learned skilled movements not attributable to elementary sensory or motor dysfunction. Four types have been traditionally described and will be mentioned briefly.

Ideomotor apraxia

Ideomotor apraxia is the inability to perform single actions. Such actions may be performed automatically, as with shaking hands on meeting friends. Thus, the inability may only be revealed if the patient is asked to demonstrate actions or to imitate the actions of the examiner. In the testing situation the patient may be asked to wave good-bye, blow a kiss or show how to use a toothbrush.

It may result from disconnection of the language area from the motor area, such that the request is comprehended but the message cannot be relayed to the appropriate area (Rosen, 1991). This does not explain cases where the patient cannot imitate the examiner.

Ideational apraxia

Ideational apraxia is the inability to perform a series of actions because of difficulty with sequencing the movements. The 'idea' of the actions is disrupted. In the testing situation the patient may be given the materials and be asked to fold a piece of paper, place it in an envelope, and then seal, address and stamp the envelope.

Most commonly this is a feature of confusional states or severe dementia, but focal callosal, left parietal and biparietal lesions may produce the sign (Ovsiew, 1992).

Constructional apraxia

Constructional apraxia denotes difficulties with 'constructions' (Mueller and Fields, 1984). Recent authors avoid the term apraxia in this context, preferring 'constructional problems' (Howieson and Lezak, 1992). In the testing situation the patient may be asked to copy a drawing on paper or an arrangement of blocks or sticks.

Posterior lesions of left or right hemisphere or diffuse brain damage may result in these problems.

Dressing apraxia

Dressing apraxia is difficulty in orienting articles of clothing with reference to the body. It has a long tradition in neurology, but is not mentioned by some recent authors. In the testing situation the patient is requested to put on articles of clothing such as a dressing gown or coat.

It is seen in dementia and right parietal lobe lesions, but is probably most common in confusional states.

Recognition of stimuli and agnosia

Agnosia is the inability to recognise stimuli, which is not attributable to impaired sensory processing, intellectual functioning, or naming ability (Rosen, 1991). It is most frequently specific to one modality.

Visual object agnosia

Visual object agnosia is the inability to recognise a familiar object that can be seen. In the test situation the patient is asked to identify objects which make no noise, such as a pen, a coin and a bandage.

It is seen in left occipital lobe lesions.

Agnosia for faces (prosopagnosia)

Prosopagnosia is the inability to recognise faces of people well known or newly introduced to the patient. Specific testing is necessary.

It is most frequently the result of bilateral lesions of the mesial occipitotemporal region.

Tactile agnosia

Tactile agnosia is the inability to recognise objects by touch. In the test situation the patient is asked to identify by touch, a key, a coin, a pen or a bandage.

It may result from unilateral or bilateral lesions.

Auditory agnosia

Auditory agnosia is the inability to recognise non-verbal acoustic stimuli. In the test situation the patient may be asked to identify the sound of keys jangling, water running from a tap, or the clapping of hands.

It is associated with unilateral or bilateral temporal lobe lesions.

Spatial agnosia

Spatial agnosias include disorders of spatial perception and loss of topo-graphical memory (Rosen, 1991). Some include spatial agnosia and constructional apraxia under 'visuospatial function' (Ovsiew, 1992). In test-ing, patients may be asked to locate significant geographical locations on an unmarked map and orient themselves in space using the available cues.

It is associated with bilateral cortical lesions.

Corporal agnosia and anosognosia

Corporal agnosia is the inability to recognise parts of the body (one form of which is finger agnosia) or that a part of the body is affected by disease (anosognosia).

Agnosia limited to finger identification may be found in left parietal lesions (in right-handed people), while anosognosia is associated with right parietal lesions.

9. Rapport

Most recent textbooks make no mention of rapport. For the sake of completeness, a brief outline is offered.

There is no widely accepted definition of rapport. In general, the term refers to a comfortable, unconstrained, mutually accepting interaction between two people. In a psychiatric assessment, it is beneficial for patients to expose their thoughts and feelings. Good rapport makes this process easier and more complete.

Rapport exists between two people – the patient and the interviewer both contribute. Both bring attributes and attitudes to the relationship, so that the transference and counter-transference issues described in psychotherapy also have importance in the assessment of rapport.

One view is that as long as interviewers behave in a respectful and professional manner, and give due consideration to their contribution to the relationship, that the examination of the quality if the rapport which is developed has diagnostic value.

Diagnostic considerations

Better-than-expected rapport

This is a little disheartening. When rapport between the patient and the clinician seems flawless, the clinician needs to be especially alert, as almost certainly, something is going wrong.

The gifted person

When better-than-expected rapport develops, consideration must be given to the possibility that one is dealing with an unusually gifted, confident person, well trained in interpersonal skills and free of mental disorder. But, such a person is unlikely to be seeking psychiatric assessment.

Mild mood elevation

One alternative may be that this individual is mildly mood elevated, and that this helps him or her to be confident, quick witted, charming, happy, flirtatious and smiling.

Personality disorder

Another possibility is that the patient has a histrionic personality disorder and is, in fact, behaving in a dramatic, seductive and dependent manner. Here the word seductive is used not in the sexual context (although that may also be the case) but in the context of persuasion away from principles of usual practice – the unusually long appointment, the discussion of mutual interests rather than the patient's problems. Such a patient may appeal to our desire to be important by saying – 'Well Doctor, you might not believe this but, I've never told this to anyone else before, but ...'. It is wise not to believe that one is special.

The early stages of the relationship with a person with a dependent personality disorder may go along similar lines.

Drug seeking behavior/malingering

Individuals seeking drugs for personal misuse or trade may attempt to establish an especially close relationship with the clinician. Once this is achieved the individual can make the clinician feel obligated and guilty if they do not help them with some 'special problem'. Malingering people may be seeking compensation, escape from responsibility or inappropriate benefits and may also seek to establish a special relationship.

Poorer-than-expected rapport

Paranoid person

It is often very difficult to establish good rapport with a paranoid person. This applies to an individual with a paranoid personality as well as a psychotic disorder. Things go better if the clinician takes particular care to be respectful and accurate in statements.

Schizoid person

The schizoid individual has less interest than usual in, or need for, interpersonal relationships. It follows that rapport is difficult to establish.

Avoidant person

The avoidant person feels socially inadequate, is hypersensitive to, and fears social rejection. Such people are socially inhibited. Naturally, it may be difficult to establish good rapport with such a person. Nevertheless, the avoidant person may have the desire to engage in a relationship and good rapport may be possible if the clinician is able to provide reassurance and support.

Schizophrenia

People with schizophrenia have difficulty establishing rapport with others. At times they are paranoid. They may be schizoid and have less than the usual interest or need for interpersonal relationships. Further, the negative symptoms make rapport even more problematic. There may be the loss of the ability to experience pleasure, lowered energy, poverty of thought and flat affect, and these disable as well as render such individuals less engaging company.

Depression

It may also be difficult to establish good rapport with seriously depressed patients. They may have psychomotor retardation and be thinking and speaking slowly. Their faces may be unsmiling, voices monotone and they may lack energy. They may be preoccupied with their own problems and show no interest in the interview or interviewer.

10. Insight

In ordinary language the word insight is synonymous with understanding. In psychology and psychiatry the word has a number of different technical applications, all of which retain that element of understanding. In psychology the term has been used to describe a form of learning (configuration) in which there is the sudden grasping of a solution.

In psychiatry insight may be broadly defined as awareness of one's own mental condition. However, there are different shades of meaning, depending on the type of disorder present and the concepts employed. Insight is an important factor in the development of the therapeutic relationship – generally, the less insight, the more difficult is the development of the therapeutic relationship (although insight is not an absolute requirement for a therapeutic relationship). Insight usually changes, at least to some extent, during the course of an episode of illness (Figure 37).

At this point, it is necessary to introduce the term, 'psychosis', which has been defined as, 'a mental disorder in which a person's mental ability, affective response, and ability to recognise reality, to communicate, and to relate to others are impaired enough to interfere with the capacity to deal with the ordinary demands of life'. Psychoses occur in schizophrenia, delusional disorder, and in some cases of mood disorder, organic mental disorder and psychoactive substance use disorder. When a patient is suffering a psychosis, it is assumed they are 'psychotic', by which is meant they have all, or most of, the symptoms of a psychotic disorder (including lack of insight). Caution is necessary. For example, it is possible for an individual to have one, or more, of the so-called psychotic symptoms and not be suffering from a psychotic disorder (anorexia is an example). On the other hand, they may be suffering a psychotic disorder with some psychotic symptoms, but not be psychotic (for example, an individual who has schizophrenia with persistent hallucinations who has insight and is able to work and function as a partner and parent). Nevertheless, the above definition of psychosis allows for a working division of mental disorders into non-psychotic and psychotic groups. The caveat is that an individual may be profoundly incapacitated by a mental disorder, but not have a

> I've been told I'm Schizophrenic
>   but I don't think I am.
> The only feelings I have   are
>   confusion, plus whether I look normal.
> I feel as if I'm being punished for a crime
>   I didn't commit,
>   . Actually I don't know who to blame, at times
> My thoughts seem to linger into each other
>   therefore I get completely confused.
> I feel so lost and lonely.
> I once heard a phrase which went, " who can
>   you tell if you haven't a friend",
> Which I am feeling very strongly, about so I decide
> -d, to write it on paper.
>   So. someone, anyone,! could you listen
>   and give me an explanation.
> Or   even maybe help sort out my confused
>   state of mind.
>
> I don't want to take heaps of tablets
> I WANT a truthful explanation to my feelings
> So that once and for all can
>   understand my mind, and why it is constantly
>   confused.

Figure 37. This was written by a twenty-year-old woman who suffered schizophrenia. Two years later she died by suicide.

This document illustrates lack of insight. It was written at a time when she was in remission, living independently and without delusions. She found the suggestion that she was suffering schizophrenia to be very threatening and distressing. There is perplexity, 'I don't know who to blame', which has at times had a paranoid flavor, 'I feel I'm being punished for a crime I didn't commit', which made insight difficult to maintain.

The patient felt 'lost and lonely'. Despite a very large amount of time spent in discussion from the full range of mental health professionals, she still felt unheard and unconvinced, 'could you please listen and give me an explanation'.

There is some derailment, but this is not pronounced. However, she found the subjective experience of thought disorder to be distressing (probably because it produced a sense of loss of control), 'My thoughts seem to linger into each other therefore I am completely confused', 'help sort out my confused state of mind' and 'understand my mind and why it is constantly confused'. (Of course a contribution for this 'confusion' may have come from disorder of content of thought, into which there was partial insight.)

psychotic disorder, or be suffering a psychotic disorder, yet still able to meet the challenges of everyday life.

The non-psychotic disorders include anxiety, somatoform, dissociative, sexual, adjustment and personality disorders. Generally speaking, patients with non-psychotic disorders have 'insight' (meaning they are aware that they have a mental disorder). In fact, the presence of insight is sometimes taken as proof of non-psychotic status.

[An apparent contradiction arises from the use of the word insight in different groups of patients – that is, those patients who have insight (non-psychotic) are often treated with 'insight-orientated psychotherapy' (the aim of which is to cure through the attainment of insight). If readers understand this sentence they understand the full range of meanings of the term.]

Insight is not an all-or-none phenomenon. It is better regarded as a matter of degree. As with other mental state phenomena, relevant information gathering on this aspect continues throughout any interview, but is incomplete without direct (albeit subtle) questioning. The following are schema for assessing insight, at a point in time, taking into account the differences between non-psychotic and psychotic disorder.

Assessing insight in non-psychotic disorders

When the non-psychotic patient is assessed, particularly one who has received insight-orientated psychotherapy, at least three levels of insight can be considered.

Minimal insight in non-psychotic disorder

When there is minimal insight in non-psychotic disorder, patients will explain their difficulties in terms of physical problems, or blame features of the external environment.

Intellectual insight in non-psychotic disorder

When there is 'intellectual insight' in non-psychotic disorder, the patient has knowledge of the disorder and understands some of aetiological factors, but this is insufficient to alter future behaviour and experiences.

Emotional insight in non-psychotic disorder

When there is 'emotional insight' in non-psychotic disorder (which is usually achieved through psychotherapy) the patient has an awareness of motives and deeper feelings and this may lead to a positive change in personality or patterns of behaviour.

Assessing insight in psychotic disorders

The following scheme may be applied in either non-psychotic or psychotic disorders, but it has greater application in the case of psychotic disorder. (Those with non-psychotic disorder are usually more aware of the presence of a disorder and the need for treatment.)

Aware/unaware of the phenomena

The first step is to determine whether the patient is aware of the phenomena other people have observed. Most psychotic people are aware of their phenomena. By definition, patients are aware of hallucinations. However, people with mood disorder may be unaware of phenomena (a manic patient may be unaware of overactivity).

If the patient does not volunteer the information, the clinician could asked, 'Have you noticed any change in yourself today, or in the last few days?'.

If the patient denies or appears to be unaware of phenomena it will be necessary to make suggestions. In the case of a patient who is lacking insight, there may be confrontation if the examiner is precise in this matter. Confrontation may be necessary at some point, but is better avoided in the early part of the assessment.

In the case of an overactive person, ask, 'The people who brought you in (or the nursing staff, etc.) are a bit concerned about you. Do you think you might be a bit overactive (or not getting enough sleep, etc.), at all?'.

Aware/unaware that phenomena are abnormal

The second step is to determine whether the patient is aware that it is abnormal to experience such phenomena. The patient with schizophrenia who is experiencing auditory hallucinations may report them, but maintain that this is a normal experience which is available to anyone who accepts the possibility. The patient with mania may admit to being more than usually active but maintain this is no more than normal high spirits.

In the case of an overactive person one may ask, 'So, let me understand, Mr X. You have noticed that you are a bit more active than usual ... But do you think you might be abnormally active, at all......?'

In the case of an hallucinating person one may ask, 'Mr Y, you've said you've been hearing a voice when there's no one nearby. Can I ask you, do you think it is normal to hear a voice when there's no one nearby?'.

Aware/unaware of mental disorder

A third step is to determine whether the person is aware that they are suffering from a mental disorder. In some cases the distinction between awareness of abnormality and awareness of mental disorder is unclear, and in such circumstances there is little point pursuing the matter at length. However, a common finding is that psychotic patients are aware of the abnormality of their experiences, but believe these to be the result of causes other than mental disorder. Paranoid people may believe they are being poisoned (an abnormal event) by enemies, while mood-elevated persons may believe they have received a blessings given by God.

This is not usually a difficult question to frame – 'Mr Z, you have this problem of being over active. Do you think you could have some sort of mental problem, at the moment?'.

In the case of a deluded person, it is still worth asking the question. Some psychotic people are able to hold two explanations simultaneously. In other cases, belief may swing backwards and forwards from one explanation to the other. Where there are delusions, it is appropriate to ask, 'Mr X, I know you believe these troubles have been caused by the KGB ... But could there be another explanation? Could it be that your suffering a mental problem, at the moment?'.

Accepting/rejecting the need for treatment

A further step in assessing insight is to determine whether the patient accepts the need for treatment. A final issue is whether the patient who accepts the need for treatment actually accepts treatment.

In the acute stage, most, but not all, of those who accept that they have a mental disorder, accept the need for treatment. While acceptance of

the presence of a mental disorder but non-acceptance of the need for treatment may reflect a limitation of insight, religious and other previously
held views will continue to influence thinking.

In chronic disorders, non-acceptance of treatment may reflect a choice
between ineffective medication with unacceptable side effects and familiar
symptoms.

Diagnostic considerations

Rarely does the presence or absence of insight determine a diagnosis –
instead, it guides thinking in one general direction or the other (non-
psychotic or psychotic). The rest of the data from the examination of the
patient are then brought into play and a precise diagnosis becomes possible.

People with personality disorder have little awareness of the contribution of their own personality to their distress or that of others. They
deny responsibility and blame the failings of others and environmental
factors. To this extent they lack insight.

Personality disorder may be associated with subjective distress for
much of the time; alternatively, distress may only occur at times of loss.
Whether or not the losses occur as a consequence of features of the personality disorder, loss is ubiquitous to the human animal and people with
personality disorder are less well equipped to deal with loss than those
with healthy personalities. People with personality disorder are aware that
they have distress and to this extent, they have insight. Insight, however,
may be rudimentary. A person with borderline personality disorder, for
example, may only be able identify their emotional experience as either
'not distressed' or 'distressed' (see entry on alexithymia). This may result
in cutting to relieve distress. (The cutting refered to here is usually lacera-
tion of the outer aspect of the forearm.)

In certain non-psychotic disorders (those designated neurotic disorders in ICD-10) there is a symptom or group of symptoms that is distressing
to the individual and is recognised by him or her as unacceptable; reality
testing is intact. Thus, insight is present and the degree may be determined
according to the schema described above.

The degree of insight into recurrent thoughts can be an important
clinical issue. Recurrent thoughts into which there is good insight and
which are recognised by patients as the product of their own mind, are
likely (depending on concurrent phenomena) to be features of the non-
psychotic, obsessive–compulsive disorder; while recurrent thoughts

believed to be inserted from outside are likely to be a feature of the psychotic disorder, schizophrenia.

It is important to know whether or not certain thoughts constitute a delusion. When a delusion is held, the patient lacks insight. Delusions about physical illness or defect indicate a psychotic disorder, whereas similar ideas which are not held with delusional conviction (into which there is insight) indicate a non-psychotic, somatoform disorder. However, the delusion that the body is overweight when this is not so (a situation in which there is lack of insight) indicates the non-psychotic disorder, anorexia nervosa, unless supported by additional psychotic symptoms.

In depressive episodes, insight has been described as 'excessive', highlighting the general tendency of depressed people to draw attention to their distress and their problems. Depressed mood may influence thinking such that the patient becomes pessimistic (refuses effective treatments because of the belief that nothing will help) and in the extreme, suffers loss of insight and delusions of guilt. In manic episodes, judgment is poor and accordingly, the patient may engage in uncharacteristic behaviour. There may or may not be delusions, but usually, there is early loss of insight.

While patients may recognise hallucinations for what they are, it is less common, if not definitionally impossible, for there to be insight into delusions. Transient delusions may occur in drug-induced psychosis and mood disorder; more permanent delusions occur in schizophrenia and delusional disorder. Where there are prominent delusions and little insight, patients are often brought for assessment by the police, friends or family. Over time, persistent delusions either become less troubling or patients learn that other people do not share their belief and draw attention to them less. In real life, many people who have suffered psychotic illness, live and function in society while experiencing residual delusions.

Management is greatly influenced by the degree of insight. Insight is desirable. It allows the individual to function more effectively, with dignity and autonomy. Thus, where insight is lacking, in general, the patient is well served by others if their activities lead to the gaining of insight. There is always the consideration that lack of insight may have a protective function, protecting the patient from the reality that they have a mental illness, and thereby, from depression. Caution may be necessary when working to increase insight. Curiously, insight is not essential for useful cooperation between the patient and the clinician. As pointed out earlier, patients as well as people without mental disorder can function in accordance with two sets of reality simultaneously.

The absence of insight may place the patient and other people in danger and is central to legislation which allows compulsory retention and treatment of patients suffering psychotic disorders.

The Frontal Lobes

The mental state examination which has been taught and used in clinical practice for generations has been described in the preceding pages. While different versions have been advanced by different authorities, the traditional mental state examination has included components of appearance, behaviour, talk, mood, affect, thought, perception, memory, concentration, orientation, intelligence, insight and rapport.

These are either observations by the examiner of patients as they present, as in appearance and talk, or observations of patients performing tasks, as in orientation and concentration. In testing, the approach has been to examine single mental functions, such as in the testing of recent memory. Due to the lack of certain knowledge, there was little attempt (in stark contrast to the associated discipline of neurology) to relate the detected clinical phenomena to pathology in particular areas of the brain.

Advances in neuroscience have revealed something of the frontal lobe functions. Phylogenetically and otogenetically, the frontal lobes are the most recently developed parts of the brain. They are involved in language and other diverse, higher-order mental processes. The frontal-subcortical circuits form one of the principal organisational networks of the brain and are involved with the integration of information. The recognition of the importance of these circuits (which include the basal ganglia and thalamus) is an important, recent step (Joseph, 1999).

Lesions of cortical–subcortical circuits at any level can disrupt functioning of the system. Thus, it is essential that the interviewer interpret results only after conducting a full examination.

Consideration of frontal lobe functioning and the testing (where tests are available) of such functions should now be considered a central part of the psychiatric diagnostic interview. In time, a convention will emerge regarding the best place in the record of interview for the results of frontal lobe testing. At present, it seems appropriate to perform and report the frontal lobe tests somewhere after memory and before insight – this remains a matter for discussion.

The purported function and any appropriate bedside or office tests of the frontal lobe areas will be described – the chapter will end with mention of the frontal release reflexes.

Precentral region

This region does not have significant psychiatric correlates, being predominantly involved in motor activity and sensorimotor integration. It is included here for the sake of completeness, and because physical symptoms may indicate generalised pathological processes in the cortex.

For descriptive purposes, the precentral region has been regarded as two transverse strips.

The primary motor cortex

The primary motor cortex or precentral gyrus (being bounded posteriorally by the central sulcus) is Brodmann area 4. Although designated a 'motor' cortex, this area is also involved with somatosensory perception. Lesions in this area of cortex or the subcortical elements of the associated circuit result in weakness and incordination.

Office tests

· Motor strength of hand grip. The patient is asked to grip the examiners fingers. Strength should be roughly equal, with greater strength on the dominant side. It should be difficult for the examiner to free the fingers.
· Motor speed, as in finger tapping, has also been listed as a useful test (Malloy and Richardson, 1994) but such tests do not discriminate from the premotor cortex.

Diagnostically, it is important to be sure the patient is motivated and co-operating. Poor performance suggest either local lesions such as vascular or neoplastic pathology, or a generalised lesion such as a degenerative disease.

The premotor cortex

The premotor cortex, which forms a transverse strip between the primary motor area and the frontal eye fields, is Brodmann area 6. It is involved in sensorimotor integration. Lesions in this area of the cortex or the subcortical elements of associated circuits cause inability to make use of sensory feedback in the performance of smooth movements and in apraxia.

Office tests

· Sensorimotor abilities are tested by having the patient touch each finger to the thumb in succession as rapidly as possible. Watch for speed and dexterity.

· Apraxia can be tested by asking the patient to 'blow a kiss' and demonstrate the use of a shovel.

Again, it is important to have cooperation. Poor performance carries the same diagnostic implications as for motor cortex above.

Frontal eye fields

The frontal eye fields, which are between the premotor area and the prefrontal lobes, are Brodmann area 8. [Some authors (Tranel, 1992) include the lateral part of Brodmann area 8 in the lateral prefrontal cortex.] Lesions do not have direct psychiatric consequences, but the area is included here for the sake of completeness and because deficits in performance suggest the presence of a pathological process.

Conjugate eye movements are those in which the eyes turn simultaneously in the same direction. Saccadic eye movements rapidly fixate a new image on the macula. Pursuit eye movements are slower and enable the image of a moving target to remain on the macula. Saccadic eye movements are generated through pathways from the frontal eye fields. Pursuit movements are controlled by pathways from the posterior parietal cortex.

In irritative lesions (focal epilepsy) of the frontal region the head and the eyes may be turned to the side opposite the lesion. In paralytic lesions (strokes and injuries) the eyes may be turned to the side of the lesion, because of unopposed stimulus from the opposite cortex (McLeod *et al.*, 1995). Such deviation is generally temporary.

Office tests

· Ask the patient to look to either side, up and down.
· Ask the patient to follow the movement of a finger from left to right and up and down.

Most frontal lobe lesions are paralytic. In the acute stage there will be deviation of the eyes to the side of the lesion. There will be difficulty with looking to the other side on command, but there will be retention of the ability to pursue the moving finger.

In Wilson's disease and Huntington's disease there may be marked slowness of saccadic movements (Adams and Victor, 1995).

Using neurophysiological technology, eye movement defects have been detected in people with schizophrenia. There have been no reports that bedside or office tests are helpful in the diagnosis of this disorder.

Dorsolateral prefrontal cortex

The dorsolateral prefrontal cortex (DLPC) is Brodmann areas 9 and 10. These form a crescent around Brodmann area 46, which is a major contributor to the dosolateral prefrontal–subcortical circuit (Mega and Cummings, 1994).

The DLPC and the associated subcortical circuit structures are responsible for executive functions. The executive functions include the integration of sensory information, the generation of a range of response alternatives to environmental challenges, the selection of the most appropriate response, maintenance of task set, sequential ordering of data, self-evaluation of performance and the selection of a replacement response if the first applied response fails.

It is the executive functions which largely determine the ability of the individual to cope with the continuous, but ever-changing challenges of the environment. Thus, the patient's ability to make an appointment and to arrive on time is valuable information. So too, is the ability of the patient to give a comprehensive account of themselves and the reasons for the consultation.

It is believed by some authors that formal thought disorder arises from a lack of executive planning and editing (McGrath, 1991). In thought disorder there are frequent examples of failure to maintain set (distractibility), sequentially order information, and to ensure that the listener is comprehending.

In general terms, lesions of the dosolateral prefrontal–subcortical circuit will result in a failure to integrate disparate sensory elements, a limited set of responses to environmental challenge, loss of goal, perseveration and lack of self-monitoring of errors (Malloy and Richardson, 1994).

Office tests

· Is the patient able to make an appointment, make the necessary arrangements and arrive on time?
· Is the patient able to give a coherent account of current problems and the reason for the interview? Is there evidence of thought disorder?
· Digit span, days of the week or months of the year backwards. Here the patient has to retain the task and the information, and then manipulate the information. The patient with a deficit may have difficulty reorganising the information and revert to saying it forwards.
· Categorical word fluency tests. The patient is asked to produce as many words as possible, in one minute, starting with F, then A, then S (Benton,

1968). Other categorical fluency tests include naming animals, fruits and vegetables (Monsch *et al.*, 1992). While generating these lists, the patient must maintain the task set: words are not to include proper nouns or be previously used words with a suffix.

For a formal result, it is necessary to test under strict conditions, using norms. However, valuable information may be obtained without formal testing. Generally, a normal individual will be able to provide more than ten items for each of these categories, while a patient with significant deficits will usually score less than eight. The performance of the task will also provide valuable information. Common errors include perseveration which takes the form of repeating words which have already been given either during the task at hand or an earlier task. There may also be inappropriate or profane utterances.

· Alternating hand sequences. These can be devised by the examiner. One example is that one hand is placed palm upwards and the other is place palm downwards, and the patient is then asked to reversed these positions as rapidly as possible.

Another example is that the backs of the hands are both placed downwards, but one hand is clenched and the other is open, then the patients is asked to close the open hand and open the closed hand and reverse the posture of the hands as rapidly as possible.

A final example is that the patient taps twice with one fist and once with the other, then after the rhythm is established, the patient is asked to change over – the fist which tapped twice now taps only once.

Patients with frontal lobe deficits usually perform very poorly on these tests, often being unable to follow the relatively simple instructions, and usually making many mistakes, including perseveration.

· Alternating graphic sequences. Alternating graphic sequences include copying sequences of different numbers of symbols, such as two squares followed by three triangles. These are drawn at the beginning of the first line and the patient is then asked to continue across the line and subsequently, down the page.

· Formal neuropsychological testing may be necessary where uncertainty remains. Commonly employed tests include Controlled Oral Word Fluency Test (Benton, 1968) and the Wisconsin Card Sorting Tests (Heaton, 1985).

Head injury and dementing illnesses may result in severe impairment of the executive functions. Schizophrenia often has thought disorder as a major feature and the executive functions tests are usually also at least mildly affected. Depressive disorder may be associated with poor performance on verbal fluency tests during the acute phase, which normalises with remission (Trichard, *et al.*, 1995).

Orbitofrontal cortex

The orbitofrontal cortex is Brodmann areas 10 and 11. It mediates empathic, civil and socially appropriate behaviour (Mega and Cummings, 1994). Much of the personality change described in cases of frontal lobe injury is due to lesions in this area. Patients may become irritable, labile, disinhibited and fail to respond to the conventions of acceptable social behaviour. (Phineas Gage was an eighteenth century identity who had survived a steel rod passing through his skull, but with marked personality change.) Similar changes may occur with lesions of subcortical element of the frontal–subcortical circuit, as with caudate damage in Huntington's disease.

Increased concern about social behaviour and contamination has been associated with increased orbitofrontal and caudate metabolism. This has been reported with lesions of the globus pallidus and in obsessive-compulsive disorder.

Office tests

· Does the patient dress or behave in a way which suggests lack of concern for the feelings of others or regard for accepted social customs.
· Sense of smell – test with coffee, cloves, etc.
· Go/No-go Test. The patient is asked to make a response to one signal (the Go signal) and not to respond to another signal (the No-go signal). The task may be made more demanding by reversing the customary meaning of signals, such as requiring a response to a red signal and no response to a green signal.

An example is to a ask the patient to tap a fist when the examiner says 'stop' and not to tap when the examiner says 'go' (Malloy and Richardson, 1994). Pathology is revealed when the patient is unable to inhibit movement when the examiner says 'go'.

· The Stroop Test (Stroop, 1935). This is a neuropsychological test which examines the ability of the patient to inhibit responses. Patients are asked to state the colour in which words are printed rather than the words themselves. The task is made difficult by presenting the name of colours in different coloured ink.

Cultural factors are important in making an observation of lack of civility, empathy and social concern. Eructation following a meal is considered good manners in some parts of the world, and people of the same race and city will have different sets of social values depending on socioeconomic status.

Obsessive-compulsive disorder in which there is excessive concern and caution is associated with increased metabolism in the orbitofrontal cortex (which may result from subcortical pathology).

When there is failure of inhibition, head injury, other destructive lesions (including dementing processes) and schizophrenia must be considered. Impulse control disorders and personality disorder, particularly of the antisocial type, may also result from failure of inhibition. Depressive disorder has been associated with poor performance on the Stroop Test (Trichard, *et al.*, 1995).

Anterior cingulate cortex

The anterior cingulate gyrus is Brodmann area 24. The anterior cingulate-subcortical circuit is believed to mediate motivated behaviour (Mega and Cummings, 1994), initiation and goal-directed behaviour (Devinsky *et al.*, 1995). Research is continuing to unravel the complexity of this area.

At present there is no office or neuropsychological test which can be recommended to measure the functional status of the anterior cingulate-subcortical circuit.

Akinetic mutism occurs with gross lesions (e.g., meningioma) of the anterior cingulate cortex. Such patients are profoundly apathetic, generally mute and eat and drink only when assisted. They do not respond to pain and are indifferent to their circumstances.

The apathy of schizophrenia and the immobility of depressive disorder may be associated with defects in this circuit.

Frontal release reflexes

The primitive reflexes are present in normal babies and disappear as the central nervous system matures. They reappear with brain damage and in some cases as a result of the ageing process. Their significance should not be over-rated. They are more important if they appear unilaterally or in younger individuals (Ross, 1985).

Grasp reflex

The hand is stroked, across the palm toward the thumb by the examiners fingers or the handle of the patella hammer.

When the reflex is present the fingers grasp or the thumb strongly adducts. The patient may be unable to release the grip.

Presence suggests contralateral frontal lobe disease.

Sucking (pout, snout, rooting) reflex

The lips of the patient are stroked with a finger or a spatula from side to middle and back again. Alternatively, the lips maybe tapped with the patella hammer.

Sucking movements with the lips suggest frontal lobe damage or bilateral lesions above the mid-pons.

Palmar-mental reflex

The palm is scratched firmly with a key or the handle of the patella hammer, from the fingers, toward the wrist. The positive response is a flicker in the skin on the ipsilateral side of the point of the chin.

This suggest contralateral frontal lobe damage, but the true value of the reflex is yet to be clearly determined.

Glabella tap

The patient is asked to close the eyes and the supraorbital ridge is repeatedly tapped. In the normal individual the orbicularis oris ceases to contract after two or three taps – in the pathological condition the orbicularis oris continues to contract with every tap. This reflex is used in the diagnosis of Parkinson's disease, but it may also occur with frontal damage of other aetiologies.

The Samuels Office Tests Of Cognition

Martin A. Samuels is a professor of neurology. In a recent presentation (Samuels, 1999) he gave a clear account of the cognitive tests he uses in the assessment of dementia. Because tests of mental functions are never perfect, criticism is always possible. The details of his recommended tests are given below without criticism – as an example of a practical approach taken by a competent, working clinician.

In the office setting there are four cognitive functions to be tested. These are arranged in an hierarchical manner because the patient who fails at one step will probably fail at subsequent levels and there may be little point in proceeding.

Level of consciousness

Consciousness is a spectrum which extends from alert to coma. When consciousness is impaired there exists a 'confusional state' and there is difficulty with 'attention'. When assessing the level of consciousness in dementia or other psychiatric disorders, the eyes are open and if there is impairment it is at the upper end of the consciousness spectrum. To test levels of consciousness one needs a test which 'requires a coherent stream of thought or action'. An acceptable test is the serial 7s test, however, the recommended test is the 'the one-tap, two-tap test.

In the one-tap, two-tap test, when the examiner taps once, the patients is to tap twice, when the examiner taps twice, the patient is not to tap at all.

Language

Language is a code by which organisms communicate. It has various forms, speech and writing being the most common. Language disorders are called aphasias. With spoken language there are the fluent aphasia and non-fluent aphasia. The fluent aphasias sound like language and have the prosody of language but they cannot be understood by the listener. The non-fluent aphasia do not sound like language there may be slurring and long silences. The patient may retain the ability to curse with clarity. This is because cursing communicates feelings rather than complex ideas that rely on different circuits.

It is recommended that spoken language be assessed by listening. If there is doubt, Samuels recommends the use of writing, and makes the point that even if there is a dense right hemiplegia, the patient who is free of aphasia should be able to write intelligibly with the left hand.

Memory

All dementias have memory disorder as feature. This is a most important and difficult function to examine. There are three levels of memory and they use different brain circuits.

Immediate (or short-term) recall

This has already been tested using the one-tap, two-tap test. (Thus, there is overlap between tests of attention and immediate recall.)

Short-term (or recent) memory

This can be tested by giving the patient a story or list of objects to remember and checking recall after a few minutes.

Long-term (or remote) memory

The point is made that as the clinician has limited knowledge of the patient's previous life, it is very difficult to assess long-term memory properly. It is recommended instead that the clinician finds out what the patient is interested in, be it sport, politics, arts, crafts and have a discussion with the patient on that topic. In this process significant long-term memory deficits should be revealed. It is further recommended that should doubt remain, the patient be referred for formal neuropsychological testing.

Visual and spatial skills

It is recommended that to test visual and spatial skills the patient be asked to draw a clock face and set the hands to a particular time. It is also recommended that the patient be asked to write a sentence about the weather and to sign their name. These latter two tasks test other functions in addition to visual and spatial skills, but the responses to the three tasks fit well together and can be placed in the patient's notes as a valuable, permanent, objective record of level of function.

References

Adams R, Victor M. (1994) *Principles of Neurology*. Fifth Edition. New York: Companion Handbook McGraw-Hill.

Andreasen N. (1979). Thought, language and communication disorders. *Archives of General Psychiatry*, 36: 1315-1321.

Benson D.(1992). Neuropsychiatric aspects of aphasia and related language impairments. In: *The American Psychiatric Press Textbook of Neuropsychiatry*, edited by S. Yudofsky, R. Hales. Washington: American Psychiatric Press, pp 311-328.

Benton A. (1968). Differential behavioural effects in frontal lobe disease. *Neuropsychologica*, 6: 53-60.

Berrios G. (1996). *The history of mental symptoms*. Cambridge: Cambridge University Press.

Berrios G, Gili M. (1995). Abulia and impulsiveness revisited: a conceptual history. *Acta Psychiatrica Scandinavica*, 92: 161-167.

Bleuler E. (1950). *Dementia praecox or the group of schizophrenias*. (translated by J Zinken, 1911). New York: International Universities Press.

Bremner J. (1999). Does stress damage the brain? *Biological Psychiatry*, 45: 797-805.

Carney R. Hong B. Kulkarni S, Kapila A. A comparison of EMG and SCL in normal and depressed subjects. *Pavlovian Journal of Biological Science*, 16: 212-216.

Cloninger C, Svrakic D, Przybeck T. (1993). A psychobiological model of temperament and character. *Archives of General Psychiatry*, 50: 975-990.

Cutting J. (1990). *The right cerebral hemisphere and psychiatric disorders*. Oxford: Oxford University Press.

Cutting J. (1992). Neuropsychiatric aspects of attention and consciousness: stupor and coma. In *The American Psychiatric Press Textbook of Neuropsychiatry*, edited by S. Yudofsky, R. Hales. Washington: American Psychiatric Press, pp. 277-290.

Davies D, Davies F. (1962). *Gray's Anatomy*. Thirty-third Edition. London: Longmans.

Devinsky O, Morrell M, Vogt B. (1995). Contributions of anterior cingulate cortex to behaviour. *Brain*, 118: 279-306.

Dorlan W. (1914). The American Illustrated Medical Dictionary. Seventh Edition. Philadelphia: W B Saunders.

Folstein M, Folstein S, McHugh P. (1975). Mini-mental state: A practical method for grading the cognitive state of patients for the clinician. *Journal of Psychiatric Research*, 12: 189.

Greenough W. (1984). Possible structural substrates of plastic neural phenomena. In *Neurobiology of learning and memory*, edited by G. Lynch, J. McGaugh, N. Weinberger. New York: Guilford Press.

Grenden J, Genero N, Price H. (1985). Agitation-increased electromoyogram activity in the corrugator muscle region: a possible explanation of the "omega sign"? *American Journal of Psychiatry*, 142: 348-351.

Hamilton M. (1974). *Fish's Clinical Psychopathology*. Bristol: John Wright and Sons.

Heaton R (1985). Wisconsin Card Sorting Test. Odessa, TX: Psychological Assessment Resources.

Horvath T. (1991). Consciousness and attention. In, *Foundations of Psychiatry*, edited by K. Davis, H. Klar, J. Coyle. Philadelphia: W. B. Saunders. pp. 53-60.

Howieson D, Lezak M. The neuropsychological evaluation. In: *The American Psychiatric Press Textbook of Neuropsychiatry*, edited by S. Yudofsky, R. Hales. Washington: American Psychiatric Press, pp. 127-150.

Joseph R (1999). Frontal lobe psychopathology: mania, depression, confabulation, catatonia, perseveration, obsessive compulsions, and schizophrenia. *Psychiatry,* 62: 138-172.

Kant E. (1909). *Critique of Practical Reason* (translation by T. Abbott). London: Longman.

Kaplan H, Sadock B. (1991). *Synopsis of Psychiatry: Behavioural Sciences, Clinical Psychiatry*. Baltimore: Williams and Wilkins.

Kaplan H, Sadock B. (1998) Synopsis of Psychiatry: Behavioral Sciences, Clinical Psychiatry. Baltimore: Williams and Wilkins.

Katsikitis M, Pilowsky I. (1991). A controlled quantitative study of facial expression in Parkinson's disease and depression. *Journal of Nervous and Mental Disease*, 179: 683-688.

McGrath J. (1991). Ordering thoughts on thought disorder. *British Journal of Psychiatry*, 158: 307-316.

McLeod J, Lance J, Davies L. (1995). Introductory Neurology. Third Edition. Oxford: Blackwell Science.

Martin R, Biedrzycki R, Firinciogullai S.(1991). Reliability and validity of the Apathy Evaluation Scale. *Psychiatry Research*, 38: 143-162.

Malloy P, Richardson E. (1994). Assessment of frontal lobe functions. *Journal of Neuropsychiatry and Clinical Neurosciences*, 6: 399-410.

Mega M, Cummings J. (1994). Frontal-subcortical circuits and neuropsychiatric disorders. *Journal of Neuropsychiatry and Clinical Neurosciences*, 6: 358-370.

Monsch A, Bondi M, Butters N. (1992). Comparisons of verbal fluency tasks in detection of dementia of the Alzheimer type. Archives of Neurology, 49: 1253-1258.

Mueller J, Fields H. (1984). Brain and behaviour. In *Review of General Psychiatry*, edited by H. Goldman. Los Altos: Lange Medical Publications, pp. 93-124.

Ovsiew F. (1992). Bedside neuropsychiatry: eliciting the clinical phenomena of neuropsychiatric illness. In *The American Psychiatric Press Textbook of Neuropsychiatry*, edited by S. Yudofsky, R. Hales. Washington: American Psychiatric Press, pp. 89-126.

Rifkin A. Phenomenology of mental disorders. In, *Foundations of Psychiatry*, edited by K. Davis, H. Klar, J. Coyle. Philadelphia: W. B. Saunders, pp. 199-207.

Coyle. Philadelphia: W. B. Saunders, pp. 199-207.

Rosen W. Higher cortical processes. In, *Foundations of Psychiatry*, edited by K. Davis, H. Klar, J. Coyle. Philadelphia: W. B. Saunders, pp. 199-207.

Ross R. (1985). *How to Examine the Nervous System*. Second Edition. Medical Examination Publishing Company: New York.

Reber A. (1985). *Dictionary of Psychology*. Middlesex: Penguin Books.

Samuels M. (1999). Dementing Illness. *Audio-Digest Psychiatry*, Volume 28, Issue 5, California Medical Association.

Shallice T. (1988). *From Neuropsychology to Mental Structure*. Cambridge University Press: Cambridge.

Shammi P, Stuss D.(1999). Humour appreciation: a role of the right frontal lobe. *Brain*, 122: 657-666.

Sifneos P. (1996). Alexithymia: past and present. *American Journal of Psychiatry*, 153 (7 Suppl): 137-142.

Silva S, Martin R. (1999). Apathy in neuropsyhiatric disorders. *CNS Spectrums*, 4 (4): 31-50.

Solovay M, Shenton M, Gasperetti C. (1986). Scoring manual for the thought disorder index. *Schizophrenia Bulletin*, 12: 483-496

Stroop J. (1935). Studies of interference in serial verbal reactions. *Journal of Experimental Psychology*, 18: 643-662.

Tranel D. (1992). Functional neuroanatomy: neuropsychological correlates of cortical and subcortical damage. In *The American Psychiatric Press Textbook of Neuropsychiatry*, edited by S. Yudofsky, R. Hales. Washington: American Psychiatric Press, pp. 89-126.

Trichard C, Martinot J, Alagille M, Masure M, Hardy P, Ginestet D, Feline A. (1995). Time course of prefrontal lobe dysfunction in severely depressed in-patients: a longitudinal neuropsychological study. *Psychological Medicine*, 25: 79-85.

West L. (1967). Dissociative disorders. In *Comprehensive Textbook of Psychiatry*, edited by A. Freedman , H. Kaplan. Baltimore: Williams and Wilkins, pp. 885-899.

Winchester S (1998) The Surgeon of Crowthorne. Ringwood, Vic.: Penguin Books.

Wing J, Cooper J, Sartorius N. (1974) *Measurement and classification of psychiatric symptoms*. Cambridge: Cambridge University Press.

Appendix
Report Outline

The aim of this book is to provide a structure and practical advice to clinicians who must conduct diagnostic interviews in psychiatry and related fields. The presentation of a report is another matter. Just as there are many ways to conduct an interview, there are many ways to present findings. This report outline may be of assistance.

The psychiatric history

Demographic data

Name

Age

Religion

Race

Marital status

Education

Housing

Presenting complaint

History of the presenting complaint

Personal history

Birth and early development

Family

School

Employment

Sexual, reproductive, cohabitation

Past medical and psychiatric history

Family medical and psychiatric history

Personality

History/Patient's view/Interview/Informants
Traits

Motivation, apathy and will

Severely apathetic/No evidence of apathy/Highly motivated

Mental state examination

Appearance and behaviour

Appearance
Behaviour

Talk

Articulation   Volume
Speed   Pressure
Pitch

Mood

Depression/Elation/Irritability/Anxiety/etc.
Subjective experience
Objective findings

Affect

Appropriate/Flat/Inappropriate/Labile

Thought

Form

Derailment/Flight/Incoherence/Neologism/Block/Perseveration, Echolalia/
Poverty of thought/Poverty of content/Illogicality

Content

Delusions/Obsessions, Compulsions/Phobias/Hypochondria/Suicidal
thoughts/Homicidal thoughts

Perception

Depersonalisation, derealisation/Delusional mood/Heightened perceptions/
Changed perceptions/Hallucinations/Illusions

Intelligence

Interview performance consistent with history

Cognition

Memory

Short term/recent/remote

Orientation

Time/place/person

Attention

Subtraction/reversing

Other congnitive functions

Language/skilled movement and apraxia/recognition of stimuli and agnosia

Rapport

Comfortable, unconstrained, mutually accepting interaction

Insight

Non-psychotic/Psychotic/Aware of phenomena/Aware of illness/Accepting treatment

Summary of main findings

Working diagnosis

Interviewer

Name
Signature
Date

Index